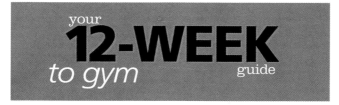

your 12-WEEK to gym guide

FROM YOUR ARMCHAIR TO A COMPLETE BODY WORKOUT IN 12 WEEKS

Fact box sources (note: conversions are from g to oz (US) and from ml to fl oz (US). (1) UK Department of Health. (2) USGS. (3) UK Department of Health. (4) UK Department of Health: Sport and Exercise Medicine: a Fresh Approach (2012). (5) McDonald's, Pizza Hut, KFC (all US). (6) P Lally, European Journal of Social Psychology. (7) US National Health Interview Survey (2010). (8) Harvard Heart Letter (July 2004). (9) Coca-Cola (US), Starbucks (US). (10) UK Department of Health: Start Active, Stay Active (2011) and US The President's Council on Physical Fitness and Sport. (11) UK Department of Health: Start Active, Stay Active (2011) and www.bootsdiets.com. (12) US National Sleep Foundation. (13) UK NHS Sport and Exercise Medicine: A Fresh Approach (2011). (14) US The President's Council on Physical Fitness and Sports: Fast Facts About Sports Nutrition. (15) Drinkaware.co.uk. (16) US The President's Council on Physical Fitness and Sports: Fast Facts About Sports Nutrition. (17) US The President's Council on Physical Fitness and Sports: Exercise and Weight Control. (18) AM Williamson and AM Feyer, British Medical Journal (2000). (19) USGS. (20) Fitness Australia. (21) *Triathlon: Serious About Your Sport* (NHP). (22) Olaf Lahl et al, University of Dusseldorf (2008). (23) JH Stubbe et al, The association between exercise participation and well-being (2006) and various others. Photos: iStockphoto.com and www. sxc.hu. P26 Alen Stojanac.P34 Robert Aichinger. P46 ayeyah. P53 Patryk Choinski, www.patrykchoinski. P56 Pawel Kryj. P59 Sanja Gjenero. P64 Peter Skadberg, www.bmmi.us. P66 Brian Lary, www.facebook. com/BrianLaryPhotography. P69 Thiago Martins, www.pubblicite.com.br. P73 Christa Richert, RGBStock. com, http://www.rgbstock.com/user/ayla87. P78-79 Nathaniel Dodson. P82 Peter Skadberg, www.bmmi. us. P88 Glenn Pebley. P91 Ramzi Hashisho. P92 Stefan Krilla, www.designticket.de. P96 Ramasamy Chidambaram, www.studiorishti.com. P102 Rodrigo Roveri, www.kzulodesign.com. P108 BSK speculator. P115 Jos van Galen. P125 Linden Laserna, www.lindenlaserna. P128 Ramzi Hashisho. P134 Matueusz Atroszko, http://atroszko.pl. P136 Matthew Bowden, www.matthewbowden.com. P141 Jos van Galen.

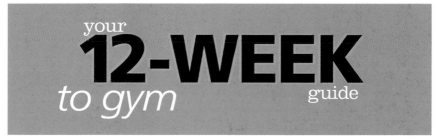

your 12-WEEK to gym guide

FROM YOUR ARMCHAIR TO A COMPLETE BODY WORKOUT IN 12 WEEKS

by Daniel Ford

Training programme by Paul Cowcher

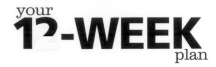

your
1**2**-WEEK
plan

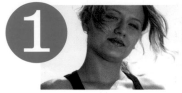

1

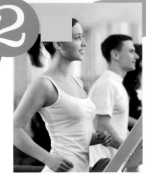

Working out

It'll be an nice easy start, but you should get ready to start working out…

Time for commitment

Simply making your mind up to go for it is a big step…

8

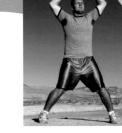

7

You're well on your way

Think back and congratulate yourself on how far you have come…

Recommit to the challenge

Picture a successful conclusion to the end of the programme…

10

9

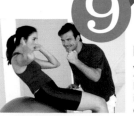

Maximize your benefit

Look at where you improve on each exercise…

Smoothly does it

Keep focused, even if things are going well at the moment…

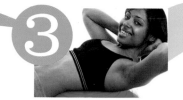

3

Rest, stretch, rest

Rest and stretching are a big part of this programme...

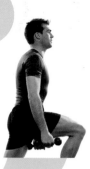

4

Workouts can be a habit

Your training sessions will soon be a part of your life...

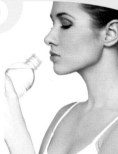

6

Soak up the fit life

You've been working hard so now you can enjoy the benefits of feeling fitter...

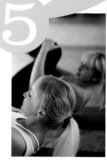

5

Nice and easy

Start to enjoy your workouts as they feel easier and smoother...

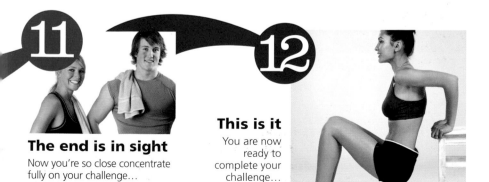

11

The end is in sight

Now you're so close concentrate fully on your challenge...

12

This is it

You are now ready to complete your challenge...

introduction

This is it, your 12-week challenge starts now...

This is the start of an exciting 12 weeks for you. You have already bought this book and made the all-important decision that you want to change things in your life. By carefully following this programme for a Complete Body Workout (see page 12) you can make positive changes. We have deliberately chosen 12 weeks because it is enough time for the programme to have a positive effect on your life but it is also a manageable chunk of time. Try to think back 12 weeks. What were you doing then? Chances are the time will have flown by. So the first thing is not to be daunted by what lies ahead.

You may have heard the question, "How do you eat an elephant?" The answer is, of course, "One bite at a time". The next 12 weeks is certainly no elephant by the way (more like a warthog) but the principle remains the same: break a large task into smaller manageable chunks and achieve them one by one to reach your end goal.

You do this subconsciously all the time in your everyday life. For instance, you don't clean your house with a single sweep of the brush. Instead

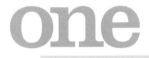

There is only one thing you should be concentrating on right now and that is to start exercising. Don't attempt to give up smoking and drinking and start eating salads just yet. You are more likely to give up if you try to change too much at once.

"The greatest achievements were at first and for a time dreams. The oak sleeps in the acorn."

JAMES ALLEN

you set about the job a room at the time; first the bathroom, then the kitchen, then the study and so on. You might even use the approach where you tell yourself, "I'll just do the bathroom, then see how I get on." The likelihood is that once you've started you carry on – but you got started only because you broke off a small chunk from the whole job that you knew you could handle. If you were to worry about the whole job all the time you'd probably let out a groan and go shopping instead.

Everyone will have their own reason for embarking on this programme. You may have had a bet with a friend who told you your best days were behind you (nothing like criticism to spur us into action, eh?). Or you may have been looking for something you can do that will help you to lose weight. Whatever your personal reason, always remember to keep focused on the goal: to follow and finish this 12-week programme for a Complete Body Workout. This is the key.

Follow the programme and the programme will look after you. Do not expect to slide into your little black dress that's become a bit too tight lately after just two workouts. Positive effects like feeling fitter, eating healthier foods and so on, are likely to happen naturally as a result of following a fitness programme correctly but don't allow them to become goals themselves. If you do this it is likely you will

hear

Listen to your body. You know when you are feeling good and you know when you are not because your body tells you. Follow the programme and listen to advice but always remember the best guide you will have is your own body.

lose motivation and stop exercising altogether. The chances of you enjoying any of the positive benefits are then zero.

Next comes the bit you might be tempted to skip. Don't. You need to spend a few seconds visualizing a successful end to these 12 weeks. We know this is strange to some people but trust us, it works. Close your eyes if it helps. Now picture yourself, feeling fitter and stronger and looking forward to your challenge. By visualizing a successful end result you are planting that success in your mind.

How to use your book

Right, now you've pictured the end result in your mind it's time to start taking the steps needed to get there. You won't need to be a rocket scientist to realize that this book is broken down into 12 large steps. Each will include a brief overview of what the focus of that particular week is all about. Read this at the end of the previous week so you've got time to digest it.

As with above, visualize the success of the week (come on, you're an old hand at this). Don't skip these few seconds of visualization as they are important in firming up the week ahead in your mind. You will also find snippets of information on things such as food and drink, mental fitness, sleep, and so on, that you can use during your 12 weeks.

see

Make sure you visualize your success before you have even taken a physical step towards it. Your mind and body work together as a team and your head is the leader so take time to picture your success right away.

The most important page in each section is Your Training Programme and Diary. Again, look over this page at the end of the previous week so the information has plenty of time to sink in. Also ensure you make space in your diary for each day's activity and don't relegate them to, "I'll fit that in somewhere," or you'll get to the end of the day and realize there is no time left. Treat each session as you would an important meeting at work or an appointment with your child's school.

At the bottom of these pages you will also see some traffic lights offering a 'Do This', 'Consider This' and a 'Don't Do This'. These are small tips that you can take on board during the week. You will also see a 'Reward' on this page, a little something to look forward to when the week is completed. Thoughtful eh? Ah, it's nothing. Use the small notes column to the right of each day to record how you're feeling. It's a great way to end a session and fun to look back on later. You will be amazed at how quickly you progress.

Finally, at the end of each chapter there is a summary of what you have achieved that week. Again, use the notes column to jot down your thoughts and feelings as this will draw a line under the week and help prepare you for the next one. Then it's time for you to give yourself a pat on the back and refer back to your reward.

when

When thinking of taking up an exercise programme for the first time or after an extended break it's important that you check with your doctor that you are fit and healthy enough. Explain your plan and get the thumbs up before starting.

Your aim this week

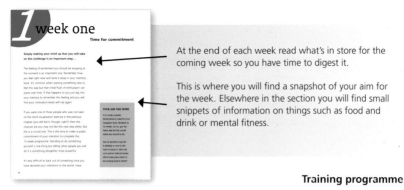

At the end of each week read what's in store for the coming week so you have time to digest it.

This is where you will find a snapshot of your aim for the week. Elsewhere in the section you will find small snippets of information on things such as food and drink or mental fitness.

Training programme

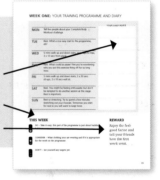

Make sure you diarize your sessions as if they are important appointments. They are.

Jot down your thoughts even if it's just, "Saw Mrs Smith as I set off for the gym. She looked impressed!" or "Felt great today".

These are additional tips you can use during your week.

This is what you are looking forward to at the end of the week.

What you have achieved

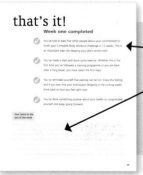

Congratulations, this is what you have completed this week.

Take a few moments to jot down your thoughts on how the week went, whether it was good or bad.

Your complete body workout target

MEN			WOMEN		
Step-ups (Heart-rate recovery test) (a)	15 bpm lower		**Step-ups** (Heart-rate recovery test) (a)	15 bpm lower	
Press-ups	20-25		**Press-ups**	7-10	
Sit-ups	30-35		**Sit-ups**	20-25	
Squats on a BOSU ball	45 secs to 1 min		**Squats on a BOSU ball**	30 to 45 secs	
Front plank	45 secs to 1 mins		**Front plank**	30 to 45 secs	

* Two minutes recovery between each exercise.

Note: these are targets for the average pizza muncher who has just decided to get out the armchair. It is possible you are particularly strong in one area of your body and you consider the target for a certain exercise too low for you. Once you have completed your trial challenge (see page 29 in Week 2) look at the targets again and decide if you want to raise the one in your strongest area. For example, if you do 28 sit-ups in the challenge when your end target is 30-35 (for a man) you may decide to raise your own challenge target. However, don't push it and remember any improvement, no matter how small, is significant. The programme is aimed at getting you fit for a Complete Body Workout not just making you a sit-up expert.

(a) Step-ups are for a heart-rate (HR) recovery test. So do step-ups for 2 mins (rough pace of each leg stepping is one per second), then take your heart rate. Have 1 min rest then take your heart rate again. Your heart rate recovery is the difference between the two heart rates. The fitter you get the quicker your heart rate will return to normal following exercise. Note: bpm = beats per minute.

Exercises

These are the exercises you will use during your 12-week programme. Read through them and make sure you are comfortable with them as poor technique will lead to wasted effort and injury. Those marked as challenge exercises are the ones you will use in your Complete Body Workout challenge at the end of 12 weeks (see page 12). The description of each exercise is the preferred method but at the end there are 'High', 'Medium' and 'Low' intensity options for each. So, for example, if you struggle with a full press-up try a press-up on a step (medium intensity). If you still struggle then try a press-up against a wall (low intensity). You will slowly build strength so you can return to the full press-up.

UPPER BODY

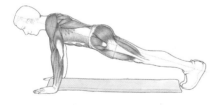

Press-ups – challenge exercise
Works: pecs, triceps, shoulders.
Start with your hands just wider than your shoulders and then lower your chest down to the floor until there is a fist-size distance between your chest and the floor. Slowly push back to the starting position. Your body should remain in a straight line – pay particular attention to the shape of your back. Keep your hips in line and then concentrate on bringing your chest down as this will keep your body straight. High: hands on floor. Medium: hands on step. Low: hands on wall.

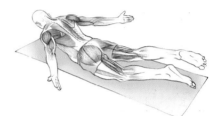

Back raises
Works: lower back.
Lie flat on your stomach, facing down, with your arms pointing away from your body (like a plane) with palms down but thumbs slightly turned up. Raise your upper body and legs off the floor so you are balanced on your pelvis. Keep your abs gently pulled in and your bum muscles gently squeezed as this will support your back. Movement up and down should be slow and controlled. High: arms out in front with your fingertips reaching out. Medium: hands by your side with your palms pointing to ceiling. Low: hands under shoulders.

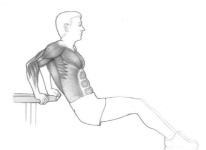

between the crown of your head, hips and heels. Back alignment is crucial and you should maintain the natural curve of your spine by keeping your pelvis centred. Pushing your weight back into your heels can really lengthen your spine. High: press-up position. Medium: leaning on elbows. Low: knees on floor.

Tricep dips
Works: triceps.

Facing away, start with your hands on a bench or step and positioned just wider than your thighs. Keep your backside close to the bench and, bending from the elbows, lower your body down towards the floor, before slowly pushing back up. Keep your shoulders pulled down all the time. At the bottom of the dip your elbows should go to a right angle and your wrists should stay in line. High: legs straight. Medium: legs bent. Low: sitting on floor.

LOWER BODY

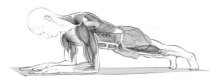

Front plank – challenge exercise
Works: abs and lower back.

To get into position place your forearms flat on the floor with your elbows just behind your shoulder alignment and your legs stretched out in a press-up position. There should be a flat line

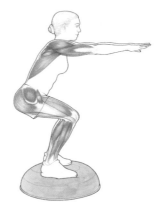

Squat on BOSU ball – challenge exercise
Works: quads, glutes, hamstrings and calves.

Start with your feet hip-width apart on the ball. Stand tall, then sit back and down keeping your back long and your chest lifted. Keep your knees in line with your middle toes. All your weight needs to be going through your heels as this will take the pressure away from your knees and activate your glutes and hamstrings. Hold this position for the time specified in the programme. High: use BOSU ball. Medium: same exercise but feet on floor. Low: feet on floor and back against a wall.

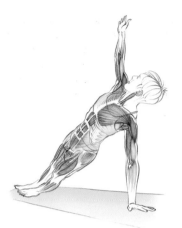

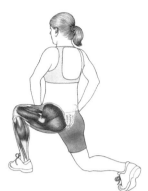

Side plank

Works: Side abs, abs and lower back.

To get into position place one hand on the floor with your elbow in a direct line under your shoulder. Your hips should be stacked one on top of the other. Then lift up as if you are drawing away from a flame until your body is diagonal to the floor. As with the front plank the key is body alignment. Your back must maintain its natural curve – lengthen your legs as this will help to keep your back long. High: Balance on feet and one hand. Low: Balance on knees (you'll have to put them at right angles).

Static lunges

Works: quads, glutes, hamstrings and calves.

With feet hip-width apart, keep your knees soft and body tall, then take a long step back, keeping your back heel off the floor. Lower your back knee down to the floor and keep your front knee in line with your middle toe. You need to keep your weight pressing through your front heel without allowing your front knee to travel forwards. Keep your pelvis gently tucked under your body. Keeping your legs in this split position raise your body so your front knee straightens, then repeat. The movement should be up and down. High: knee to floor. Medium and low: don't go as low.

Stepping alternate lunges

Works: quads, glutes, hamstrings and calves.

As with static lunge except you return your back leg to the starting position and repeat exercise with alternate legs rather than staying in the split position. High: back knee to floor. Medium and low: don't go as low.

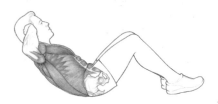

so you create a 'V' shape with your body, then lower down. The movement should be controlled and slow. As you lower yourself make sure you have full control of your body. High: raise body and legs together. Medium: bend your knees as you come up. Low: keep your feet on the floor and raise only your body.

Sit-ups – challenge exercise
Works: abs.
Lie on your back with your feet flat on the floor and your knees bent. Lightly support your head with your hands but do not pull your neck. Using your abs lift up your upper body so your shoulder blades come off the floor to about 45 degrees. Lift through your upper body and not your neck. The key is getting your shoulder blades off the floor with your eyeline looking through your knees at the highest point. To get the best results keep pulling your belly button gently back towards your spine. High: pull up to 45 degrees. Medium and low: don't pull up as high.

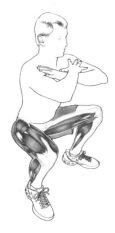

Squats
Works: quads, glutes, hamstrings, lower back and calves.
Keep your knees soft and gently squeeze your abs and bum. Tip your hips back as if you are sitting back in a chair, then go down until your legs are parallel to the floor. Push back up to the start position. Keep all your weight driving through your heels as this will maximize the workload in your glutes and hamstrings. Make sure your back stays long and keep your knees over your middle toes. If you struggle to balance, place your hand on something like a wall or table but do not let it take any weight. High: lower legs till they are parallel to floor. Medium and low: don't go as low.

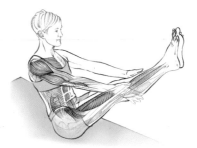

Leg raises
Works: upper abs.
Start on your back with your hands by your side. Lift up your legs and upper body at the same time

CARDIO

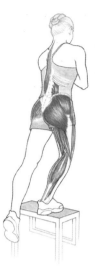

Step-ups – challenge exercise
Works: quads, glutes, hamstrings and calves.
Stand about 30 cm (12 inches) away from a step or bench. Step one foot up before bringing your other leg up, always keeping your foot and knee at a right angle. When stepping onto the bench with your first leg carefully put your heel down. This will keep your body secure on the bench and activate the correct muscles. Always keep your body straight and tall. Avoid the temptation to lean forward from your hips. High: Hold weights. Medium and low: use a lower step.

Jumping jacks
Think classic army movie exercise. Start with legs together and arms by your side. Take a small jump straight up and as you do move you legs apart (they should land apart) and at the same time swing your arms up above your head into a clap. Take another small jump and return arms and legs to their starting position. High: swing arms to a clap. Medium and low: tap arms on side rather than above your head.

Plus... Jog with knees up • Walk • Walk up and down stairs

Notes: Exercises to 'max' means you should do the most you can do until you feel poor technique occurring due to fatigue.

• Exercises with weights can be done with dumbbells, bottles of water, resistance bands, cans of food, or anything else heavy you can hold.

• The programme gets progressively harder and some exercises (eg. plank) are very challenging. If you feel light-headed or sick during or immediately after the exercise then choose another exercise from the programme that works that part of the body.

• Intensity levels on cardio exercises should be done at a maximum of 80 per cent effort. Don't go flat out.

• Rest between exercise should be between 30 secs and 1 min, except test days where you should allow 2 mins between exercises for a better recovery.

1 week one

Time for commitment

Simply making your mind up that you will take on this challenge is an important step...

The feeling of excitement you should be enjoying at the moment is an important one. Remember how you feel right now and store it away in your memory bank. It's common when starting something new to feel this way but that initial flush of enthusiasm can wane over time. If that happens to you just dig into your memory to remember this feeling and you will find your motivation levels will rise again.

If you were one of those people who was not keen on the short visualization exercise in the previous chapter (you still did it, though, right?) then the chances are you may not like this next step either. But this is a crucial one. This is the time to make a public commitment of your intention to complete this 12-week programme. Deciding to do something yourself is one thing but telling other people you will do it is something altogether more powerful.

It's very difficult to back out of something once you have declared your intentions to the world. Have

YOUR AIM THIS WEEK

Is to make a public declaration to train for your Complete Body Workout in 12 weeks. Go on, get out there and tell the world what you intend to do.

You've decided to go for it already so now is the time to share it. After all, once you've told everyone about your plans there is no turning back is there?

"The achievement of your goal is assured the moment you commit yourself to it."

MACK R DOUGLAS

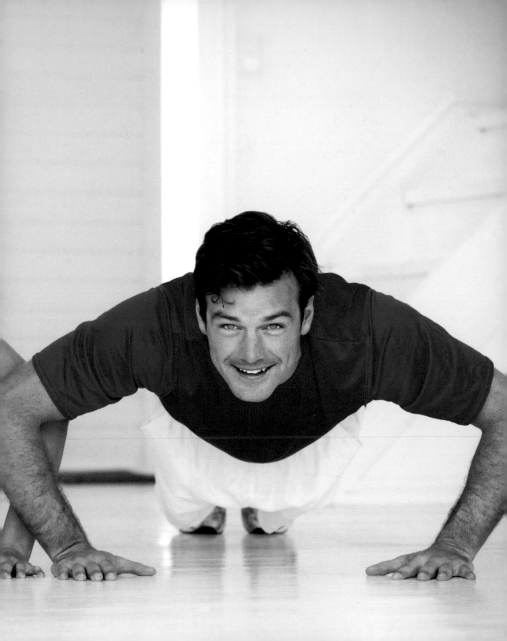

WEEK ONE: YOUR TRAINING PROGRAMME AND DIARY

		YOUR DAILY NOTES
MON	Tell five people about your Complete Body Workout challenge.	
TUE	Rest. What a nice easy start to the programme, eh?	
WED	5 mins walk up and down stairs, press-ups to max, 3 x 10 secs front plank.	
THU	Rest. What could be easier? Bet you're wondering why you put this exercise thing off for so long now.	
FRI	5 mins walk up and down stairs, 2 x 20 secs sit-ups, 3 x 10 secs squat on BOSU ball.	
SAT	Rest. You might be feeling enthusiastic but don't be tempted to do another session at this stage. Rest is important.	
SUN	Rest or stretching. Try to spend a few minutes stretching out your muscles. Tomorrow you start for real so you will want to keep loose.	

THIS WEEK

 DO – Take it easy; this part of the programme is just about building habits.

 CONSIDER – What clothing your are wearing and if it is appropriate for the work on the programme.

DON'T – Worry you won't be able to get to the end goal as there is plenty of time.

REWARD

Enjoy the feel-good factor and tell your friends how the first week went.

you ever seen someone who has proudly announced to the whole office that they are giving up smoking for good only for you to see them having a sneaky puff out the back a few weeks later? They look a bit sheepish don't they? That's because none of us likes to fail or, just as importantly, none of us likes to show others that we have failed or don't have the will to succeed. It's a feeling that actually stops a lot of people sharing their dreams with others, or worse still, stops some dreaming altogether. Ah, but we can tell by your fine choice of reading material that you are not one of these people.

So now is the time to tell at least five friends, family or colleagues at work about your plan. This is the first day of your training programme and you wouldn't want to be skipping your first day now, would you? Try to do this face-to-face (or at least on the phone if someone you want to share it with lives a fair distance away from you). If it's less daunting then you can send an e-mail or post a message on Facebook but the commitment effect will be much stronger if you do this in person.

Make sure you tell some people who you feel certain will support your fitness plans (who knows they may even join you over the next 12 weeks?). But as word spreads expect apathy from some, which is difficult to understand when you are so pumped up about something. But, hey, each to their own. And

20

Is the number of minutes you will be exercising this week. This is probably less than the time you might spend having a coffee with a friend or even watching your favourite television programme. Not a lot when you think of it like that is it? Make sure you find the time for exercise just as you would any other activity.

"The irony of commitment is that it's deeply liberating – in work, in play, in love."

ANN MORRISS

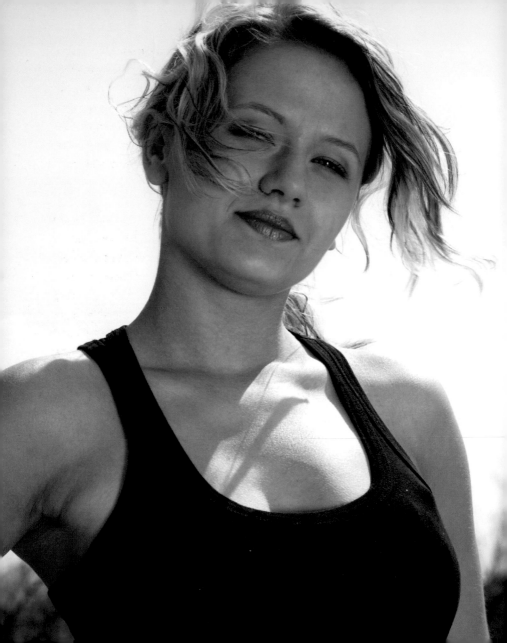

Women doing enough exercise

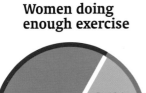

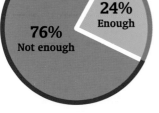

24%
Enough

76%
Not enough

Only 24 per cent of women (37 per cent of men) in the UK do enough exercise according to government health guidelines. Well done, you are on your way to joining the minority!

The figures show just how easy it is for most people to fall into the trap of not keeping fit. Remind yourself of this if you ever feel like giving up in the coming weeks. (1)

chances are you are not that interested in the stamp collection that person keeps going on about either. Other people may even actively put down your plan or laugh at the idea. Do not let them put you off but use 'proving them wrong' as another thing to spur you on. Most negative responses come from those who aren't capable or determined enough to do something themselves anyway.

Once the hurdle of day one is cleared you have just two workout days (Wednesday and Friday) and you will have completed week one. Each workout includes a short walk to warm-up and a couple of easy exercises to get your muscles used to working out again. The workouts on these days will last just a few minutes in total but this is really just about getting you active after a break from exercising (has it really been that long?).

Even the most inactive people have to do some sort of exercise in their daily life, even if it is just walking to a bus or housework. All of these activities contribute to keeping you fit and healthy, so shouldn't be dismissed, but this week you have introduced some 'planned' exercise into your life, which is important from a commitment point of view and as a way of feeling good. By setting aside a few dedicated minutes for these easy sessions you are declaring that getting fit is important to you. Welcome to the start of your Complete Body

"A shortcut is the longest distance between two points."

ANON

that's it!

Week one completed

✓ You've told at least five other people about your commitment to finish your Complete Body Workout challenge in 12 weeks. This is an important step. No keeping your plans secret now!

✓ You've made a start and done some exercise. Whether this is the first time you've followed a training programme or you are back after a long break, you have taken the first steps.

✓ You've reminded yourself that exercise can be fun. Enjoy this feeling and if you ever find your enthusiasm dropping in the coming weeks think back to how you feel right now.

✓ You've done something positive about your health so congratulate yourself and keep going forward.

Your notes at the end of the week

2week two

You are ready to start working out

It will be nice and easy to start with but get ready for your workouts...

Everything up to this stage has been about preparation. You should have thought through what lies ahead and prepared yourself mentally for the upcoming weeks. You should also now be used to making time for exercising and have had a couple of nice, gentle sessions to loosen up your limbs. Now is the time to seriously get to work on the physical side of things.

The first thing to do is to become familiar with the various exercises you will be using as you train towards your Complete Body Workout (see pages 12-15). We have chosen to use a small number of exercises in this programme to keep things simple, but together they will be effective in building up strength in your upper body, lower body and your core. There are also a variety of exercises to help you build up your cardiovascular fitness.

Some of the exercises target specific areas of your body (eg. sit-ups will work your abs) while others

YOUR AIM THIS WEEK

Is to accept that you should not do more than the programme sets out – even if your enthusiasm is sky high at the moment.

The best way to reach your end goal is to slowly build your fitness and confidence. People who do too much at the start are often nowhere to be seen at the end.

"What is not started today is never finished tomorrow."

JOHANN VAN GOETHE

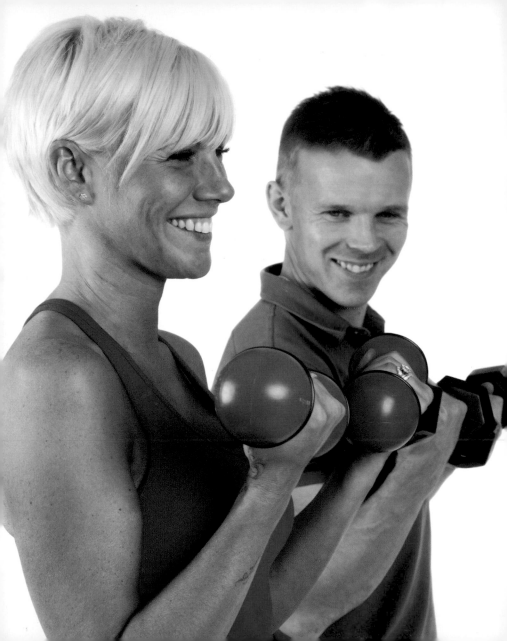

WEEK TWO: YOUR TRAINING PROGRAMME AND DIARY

		YOUR DAILY NOTES
MON	Trial challenge: All to max and with 2 mins recovery. 1 x step-ups for HR recovery test, 1 x press-ups, 1 x sit-ups, 1 x squat on BOSU ball, 1 x front plank.	
TUE	Rest. Enjoy a day off.	
WED	5 mins brisk walk, 2 x 10 tricep dips, 1 x side plank to max (both sides), 2 x 20 squats.	
THU	Rest. Consider a bit of stretching when you get the opportunity but make sure your muscles are warm.	
FRI	5 mins brisk walk, 2 x 10 tricep dips, 1 x side plank to max (both sides), 2 x 20 squats.	
SAT	Rest.	
SUN	Rest or stretching. Stretching is as much to get loose for the next day as it is to ease the muscles from exercise.	

THIS WEEK

 DO – Plan your week in advance and make sure you know what days and time you are training.

 CONSIDER – Your water intake (keeping your body hydrated is imporant). Try to have two extra glasses of water a day.

DON'T – Panic if you miss a day; the programme is flexible so you can switch rest and training days around.

REWARD

Block out an hour to yourself, put your feet up, relax.

will have you working a number of different muscles at the same time (eg. squats will work your glutes, quads, hamstrings and your lower back). You will soon discover your favourite exercises and those which you may dread (because you find them tough) but stick with the programme because it is the combination of exercises which will build your overall strength and fitness so you are ready for your challenge at the end of the 12 weeks.

You will be familiar with many of the exercises (eg. press-ups and sit-ups) but read the guidelines on how to do them carefully and make sure you are comfortable with each exercise. This is important for getting the maximum benefit from each exercise and also for avoiding injury. If you ever find yourself losing form with any exercise (eg. pulling yourself up from the neck and not your abs with sit-ups) you should stop. The programme has also been devised so that no weights and equipment are needed, so it is possible to follow it at home as well as in the gym. If you want to use weights but don't want to buy them yet then you can use bottles of water or tins of beans as substitute weights.

If you don't like people watching you when you are exercising (you are not alone by the way) then working out at home could be the ideal option. However, using a gym can give you that extra kick of 'having done something' and you may find

2.4 litres

Every day you need to replace 2.4 litres (five pints) of water that is lost or expelled from your body. Although some will come from the food you eat it's important that you drink plenty of water during the day to ensure you do not become dehydrated. (2)

"The greatest amount of wasted time is the time not getting started."

DAWSON TROTMAN

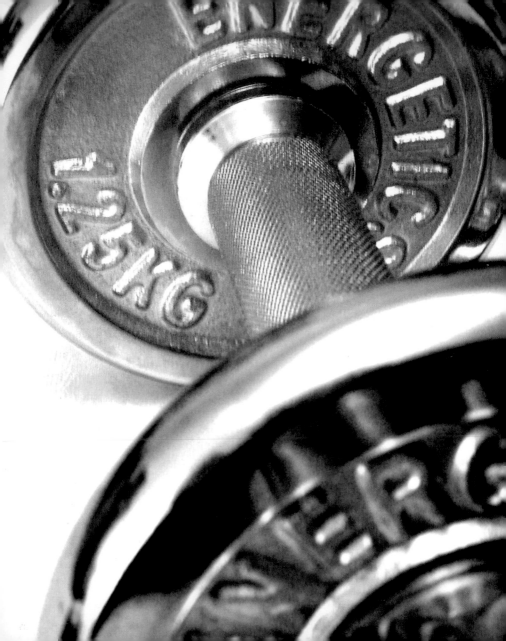

Daily calorie intake

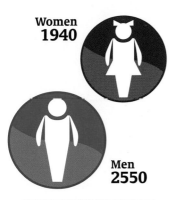

Women
1940

Men
2550

There is no need to get calorie obsessed but nutritional values are clearly marked on most food we buy so it's easy enough to keep an eye on your intake.

What you need per day depends on various factors such as your height, weight and your lifestyle. The chart shows the estimated averages by UK authorities. (3)

having other people around helps with your own motivation. As you workout more you will gain in confidence and become less self-conscious but try not to worry as most people in gyms are more worried with how they look than how others look (just see how many people are really using the mirrors to check their technique!).

This week starts with a trial challenge where you run through all the exercises in your Complete Body Workout challenge. This is partly to get you used to the exercises themselves but more importantly is to gauge your starting point. Each exercise should be done to the max (ie. until you lose technique or you simply can't do anymore) and you should rest for two minutes between each one. Don't worry if you can only do one press-up. Do your press-up, have a rest for two minutes and then move on to see how many sit-ups you can manage.

Remember this is just the starting point, so if you struggle don't get discouraged, because you have many weeks of improvement ahead of you. If you find you are super strong at one exercise then good for you. So if, for instance, you can do 18 sit-ups already when your end target is 20-25 (for women) then you may consider raising your challenge target for that particular exercise. However, don't overdo it and remember the programme is aimed at improving your overall fitness.

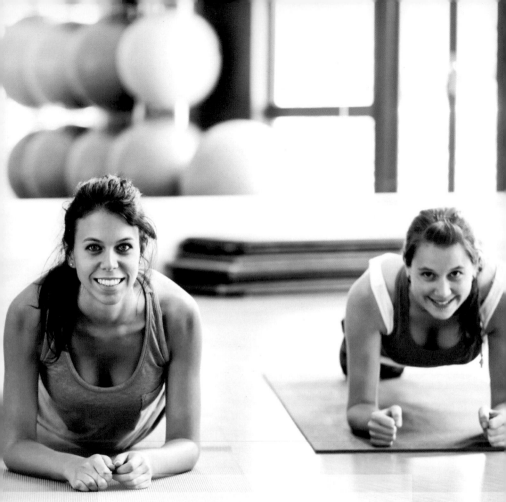

"One foot is short,
One inch is long."

QU YANG

that's it!

Week two completed

 You realize you need to follow the guidelines on how to do each exercise correctly to get the maximum benefit from it and to help avoid injury.

 You realize some people will look at you when you exercise. Workout at home if this bothers you.

You have completed a trial challenge of all the exercises that you will do in the Complete Body Workout at the end of the programme.

You've now know where you are starting from in relation to the Complete Body Workout target. Don't get discouraged if you struggled as there is still a lot of time for improvement.

Your notes at the end of the week

3week three

Rest, stretch, and rest some more

Resting and stretching, and plenty of it, are an important part of this programme...

Some people find it easy to relax while others struggle to sit still for a minute. If you find it easy to relax then good for you because rest is an important part of all fitness programmes. If you are one of those fidget pants then you're going to have to work on getting the rest part of the programme right.

Rest is important because whenever you exercise you are putting your body under physical stress. You are essentially pushing your muscles to do a bit more than they are used to, so they require the rest periods to repair themselves. Once rested properly your body will be ready for the next session. You are then able to push yourself a little bit harder the next time and, by repeating the process, build your muscles further.

Over the next few weeks you will be repeating this over and over again – pushing your body a little bit harder than it is used to then resting so it can recover. Slowly but surely the level of your

YOUR AIM THIS WEEK

Is to understand the importance of rest days. Now rest can't be difficult can it? Rest days are when your body recovers and rebuilds after exercise so treat them with respect.

You also need to be trying to get a good sleep and to be getting into the habit of stretching out your muscles before and after exercise.

"Stress should be a powerful driving force, not an obstacle."

BILL PHILLIPS

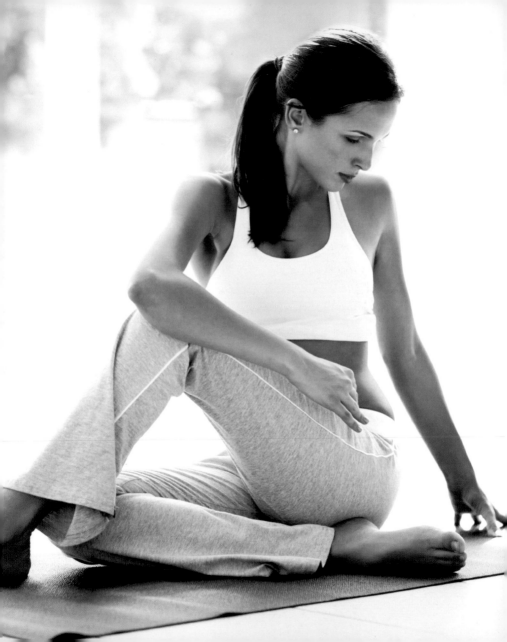

WEEK THREE: YOUR TRAINING PROGRAMME AND DIARY

		YOUR DAILY NOTES
MON	5 mins brisk walk, 2 x 10 tricep dips, 2 x 10 sit-ups, 2 x 20 squats.	
TUE	Rest.	
WED	10 mins walk up and down stairs, 2 x 10 back raises, 3 x 15 leg raises, 10 x static lunges (each leg).	
THU	Rest. Hopefully you are now getting into the habit of stretching on your rest days, even if it is just for a few minutes.	
FRI	5 mins brisk walk, 2 x 10 tricep dips, 3 x 10 sit-ups, 2 x 20 squats.	
SAT	Rest. Enjoy a nice, relaxing weekend.	
SUN	Rest or stretching. Remember to look ahead to next week and schedule in your training days to your phone or diary.	

THIS WEEK

 DO – Start thinking about your posture while exercising.

 CONSIDER – Including fruit into your food choices. Fruit can give you a natural energy boost when you need it.

DON'T – Push the intensity so hard you start losing form while you are exercising.

REWARD

Book a massage.

fitness will improve, with the eventual goal being, of course, to be ready to successfully finish your Complete Body Workout.

It's unrealistic to expect to spend the whole day totally relaxing (unless you have a very kind boss who doesn't mind you snoozing at your desk) but try to set aside some time for calmer activities you enjoy such as reading or watching a film. Things like digging the garden on your rest day is probably not the best way to help your body recover. If you really can't sit still then try to do something that is low intensity like ironing.

Now on to the king of rest: sleeping. We all know how we feel the next day if we've had a bad night's sleep. And most of us know that it's almost impossible to function properly the next day if we've worked or partied through the night. Your body is probably going to want more sleep as you start to exercise so, as much as your lifestyle permits, try to get into a regular sleeping pattern over the next few weeks. It is better to get a regular amount of sleep every night than pushing yourself to the limits at times, then trying to have a night or two where you 'catch up'.

Something else your body will be crying out for as you exercise more is stretching. This is especially true in the early days of a fitness programme because your

38%

Unless you're a particular fan of hospital food, being inactive doesn't really hold much appeal. UK research has found that inactive people spend 38 per cent more days in hospital than active people, visit their doctor 5.5 per cent more and use specialist services 13 per cent more. (4)

"Champions are not made in gyms. Champions are made from something they have deep inside."

MUHAMMAD ALI

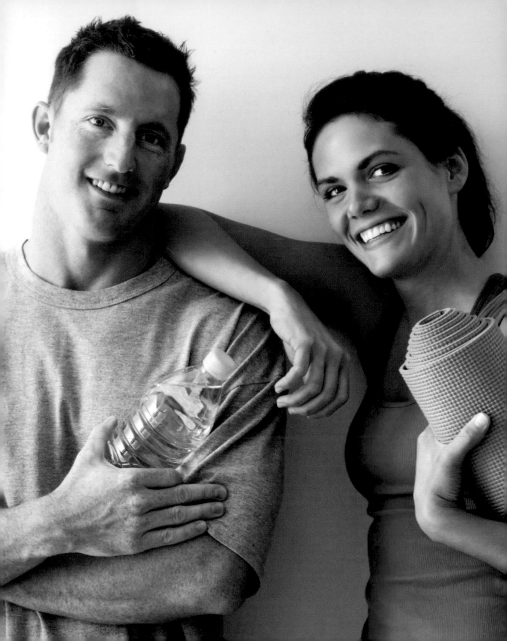

muscles will be doing things they have not done for a long time. This will lead to tightness and stiffness (as your muscles contract) and the best way to alleviate this is to stretch them out.

A lot of people skip stretching because they are too eager to get going with their 'proper' workout and don't consider stretching important enough. However, it is crucial you incorporate stretching into your programme. Just a few minutes spent loosening up your muscles at the start of a session, and again to help them cool down afterwards, will have a huge impact on the results you see. Tight, stiff muscles simply do not perform to their maximum potential. It's likely that if you haven't been exercising for a while then you haven't been stretching either, so remember to take things very gently at the start, especially when your muscles will be cold.

You should also try to get into the habit of stretching on your rest days. Even if you can only find a few minutes at the start or the end of the day (stretching is especially effective after a hot bath) you will soon start to feel the benefits of looser muscles. In fact there are always spare moments during the day – on the train, sitting at your desk – when you can stretch out certain muscles. Granted, you can't have a proper session but it's easy enough to roll your neck and shoulders while taking a rest from the computer.

Calories in takeaways

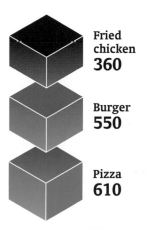

Fried chicken
360

Burger
550

Pizza
610

Nothing beats a tasty takeaway, but keep an eye on the calories. The chart above refers to a Big Mac (215 g, 7.6 oz), a Pizza Hut Pepperoni 6-inch (15 cm) Personal Pan Pizza, a KFC chicken breast (163 g, 5.8 oz). (5)

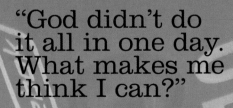

"God didn't do
it all in one day.
What makes me
think I can?"

ANON

that's it!

Week three completed

 You realize rest days are an important part of this programme. You push your muscles beyond what they are used to and the rest days are when they recover and prepare for the next session.

 You know a regular sleep pattern is important, especially when you are exercising. It is better to let your body get into a steady rhythm than try to 'catch up' on sleep.

 You are spending a few minutes before and after you exercise to stretch out your muscles.

 You know a bit of stretching on your rest days will help your muscles stay loose for the next training session.

Your notes at the
end of the week

4 week four

You workouts can become a habit

Before you know it your training sessions will be a part of your life...

Habits are formed by doing the same thing over and over again. The habits you may have formed of working too many hours, getting out of shape, and eating takeaways, didn't happen because you woke up one day and decided they would be a good idea. They probably became habits because you were tired and pressed for time, so you kept doing these things again and again until you stopped thinking about them anymore.

But the good news is that it is just as easy to form good habits as well. It's simply a matter of starting to do something you want to do and to keep doing it. You are already well on the road with exercising because you have got this far. It's now just a matter of keeping it going. The time it takes to form a habit varies from person to person, but one day you will look back and realize you've cracked it because you'll have got out of bed, pulled on your gym kit and headed off for your workout without even thinking about it.

YOUR AIM THIS WEEK

Is to keep going knowing that by doing so you are making exercise a habit in your life.

Good habits, the same as bad habits, are created simply by repeating the same action. Before you know it you will be pulling on your training gear as if it is second nature.

"Rigid, the skeleton of habit alone upholds the human frame."

VIRGINIA WOOLF

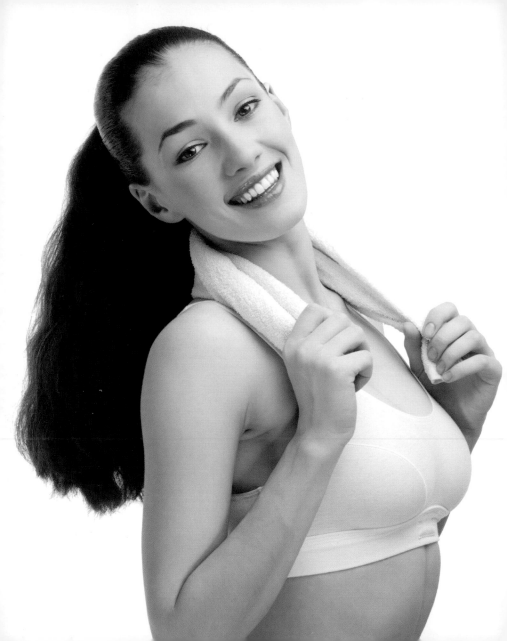

WEEK FOUR: YOUR TRAINING PROGRAMME AND DIARY

		YOUR DAILY NOTES
MON	5 mins brisk walk, 1 min jumping jacks, 2 x 15 back raises, 1 x front plank to max, 1 x 12 static lunges (each leg).	
TUE	Rest.	
WED	10 mins up and down stairs, 2 x press-ups to max, 2 x 12 sit-ups, 1 x squat on BOSU ball to max.	
THU	Rest.	
FRI	5 mins brisk walk, 1 min jumping jacks, 2 x 15 back raises, front plank to max, 1 x 12 static lunges (each leg).	
SAT	Rest.	
SUN	Rest or stretching.	

THIS WEEK

 DO – Eat something nutritious within 20 mins after finishing exercise, even if it is something small like a piece of fruit.

 CONSIDER – How many caffeine drinks you are having per day. Drinking caffeine too close to bedtime could disrupt your sleep.

DON'T – Lose motivation if results aren't instant. The results will come if you stay focused on the programme.

REWARD

Have a cheat day. Eat whatever you like and don't do any exercise. Enjoy.

There are a number of things you can to do to ensure you get to that day. Firstly you need to continue to schedule your exercise sessions into your diary or your phone so each one is marked down in the same way as an important appointment.

Don't be tempted to cancel the session just because someone rings up for a chat or it's raining and you might get wet on the way to the gym. If this is important to you – and we assume it is or you wouldn't have got this far – then continue to guard the time you have set aside for your workout as your own (although obviously there will be work and family emergencies that will take priority sometimes).

You can help with this process by looking ahead in the programme and scheduling in sessions for more than one week at a time. Many people who are training for something specific will mark all their sessions into their diary at the start of the programme to help with their planning. In that way if someone e-mails you and asks to meet up a couple of weeks down the line you don't double book at the expense of your training session.

However, if you do find yourself missing the occasional session don't let it worry you too much because you have to accept that daily life takes over sometimes. Try to avoid missing too many sessions, though, or the process of creating a habit will be broken.

66days

It takes an average of 66 days to form a habit. Although this is the average time it takes to turn something new into automatic behaviour a habit can form quicker for some or take considerably longer for others – so stick at it and exercise will soon become a habit for you. (6)

"Things start out as hopes and end up as habits."

LILLIAN HELLMAN

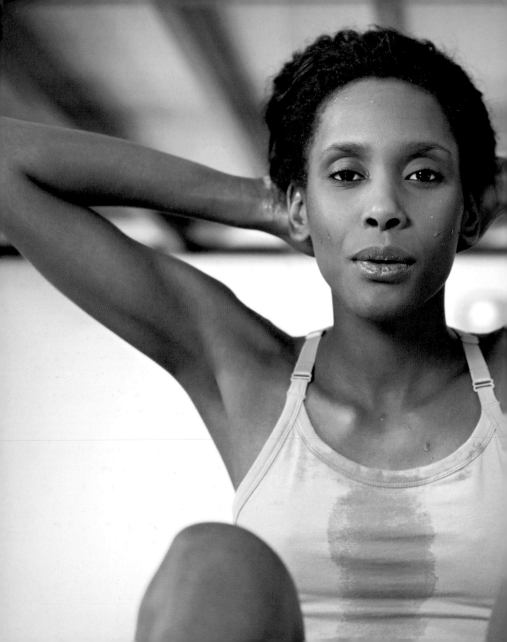

How many people get enough sleep?

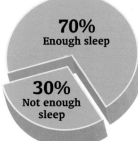

70%
Enough sleep

30%
Not enough sleep

Thirty per cent of working adults do not sleep enough (defined as less than six hours on average per day) according to a US survey.

A lack of sleep is associated with various health problems and makes it particularly difficult to train hard and get fit so make sure your lifestyle allows you to be part of the 70 per cent. (7)

One of the best things you can do is slot in your session to a time of the day you know you are least likely to be disrupted. Do you have a boss who loves to pile up your desk with paperwork just before noon and wants it sorted out as soon as possible? Then lunchtime sessions probably aren't the best for you. Three young boys that need getting ready for school? Mornings are no good then. But maybe you always have a couple of hours free after dropping the children off at school? Or you finish work early and have some time to yourself then? Some people like working out early in the morning, others after work and some when the family is tucked up in bed. Find the time that works best for you.

Remember to have some flexibility around changes in your life. If you prefer early-morning sessions but suddenly the boss calls a crack-of-dawn meeting for Wednesdays, then be prepared to shift your session to lunchtime or after work on that day.

One of the best ways to keep going is to find a training buddy. It's easy enough to wake up, decide you feel tired and go back to sleep instead of the gym when you are training solo. That's not so easy to do when you have a friend waiting outside to meet you. Training buddies are also great at motivating each other. There will always be days when one of you will be feeling a bit flat – and that's when a smile and a word of encouragement can come to the rescue.

"How we spend our days is, of course, how we spend our lives."

ANNIE DILLARD

that's it!

Week four completed

 You are gradually forming the good habit of exercising and wiping out your sit-in-the armchair habits of before.

 You are determined to keep working towards forming your exercise habit as you understand that all actions take time to become habits.

You are starting to treat your training sessions as you would any other important appointment by scheduling them into your diary. They should not be missed on a whim.

You plan your training sessions at a time of the day when you are least likely to be disrupted but at the same time need to remain flexible for unexpected life changes.

Your notes at the end of the week

week five

Nice and easy does it

You can really start to enjoy your workouts as they feel easier and smoother…

When you started training a few weeks ago you probably felt stiff and awkward. It's not surprising really, after all those months (or was it years?) of inactivity. Your poor old joints and muscles had got used to their easy life, then you started reading this book and bingo, they are dragged back into action once again.

But the great thing about your body is that it has a good memory. It might be a long time ago, but it remembers the days when it was strong and healthy. It might moan a bit at first but then, like a reluctant friend who you've asked to help you move house, it eventually mutters, "Oh, alright then", and simply gets on with the job.

Your body is also pretty good at adapting. And when it comes to exercising it adapts very quickly, especially in the early days. Right now your body is adapting rapidly and that means you are getting fitter rapidly. In fact the more unfit you were to start with, the

YOUR AIM THIS WEEK

Is to ensure that you remain loose and relaxed when you are working out.

It is not necessary to get caught up in the technical and scientific details of technique at this stage. Concentrate on keeping your mind focused on the part of the body you are working with each exercise and feel it working with each repetition.

"Happiness lies,
first of all, in health."

GEORGE WILLIAM CURTIS

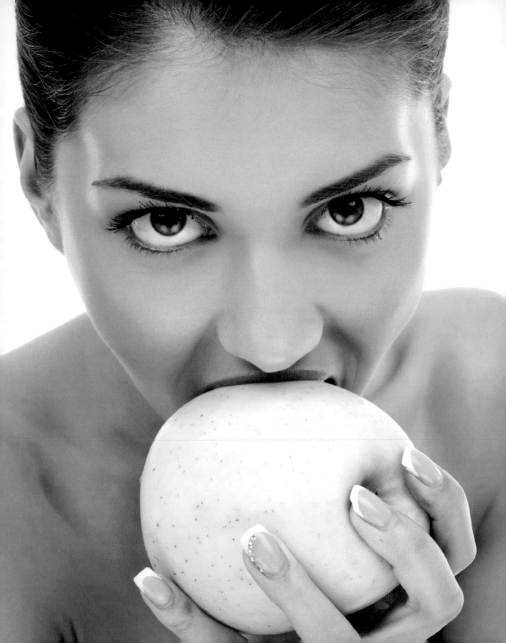

WEEK FIVE: YOUR TRAINING PROGRAMME AND DIARY

		YOUR DAILY NOTES
MON	10 mins up and down stairs, 1 min jog on spot, 2 x press-ups to max, 3 x 10 leg raises, 2 x squat on BOSU ball to max.	
TUE	Rest. Days off are even better when you feel like you deserve them, eh?	
WED	10 mins stairs, 1 min jacks, 2 x tricep dips to max, 1 x front plank to max, 1 x 20 stepping alternate lunges.	
THU	Rest.	
FRI	10 mins up and down stairs, 1 min jog on spot, 2 x press-ups to max, 3 x 10 leg raises, 2 x squat on BOSU ball to max.	
SAT	Rest. Remember your rest days are important so don't be tempted to do extra sessions.	
SUN	Rest or stretching.	

THIS WEEK

DO – Start to evaluate how you feel about the programme. If you feel you are struggling then go back and repeat a week.

CONSIDER – Healthier meat options. Try replacing red meat with white meat, or eating fish twice a week.

DON'T – Start comparing yourself to others. Focus on your own goals.

REWARD

Treat yourself to some new exercise kit.

faster you will be improving. A silver lining in just about everything, eh?

One of the most noticeable things at this stage should be the improvement in the smoothness – or the rhythm – of your movements when you are working out. Your body has slowly been getting used to the particular movements needed for each exercise which means you are becoming more efficient. Simply put, the best way to get better at the exercises in this programme is to do them and keep doing them. So stick at it and allow your body to adapt and adjust itself to what is needed. However, even though you should trust your body, it is important you are doing the exercises correctly.

Doing each exercise correctly means you will be getting the maximum benefit from them, and after all, isn't that why you embarked on this 12-week Complete Body Workout challenge in the first place? As you lose your form the benefit you gain will decrease and at worst you will be simply wasting your time and heading for an injury.

Re-read and familiarize yourself with the instructions for each exercise on pages 12-15 and keep focused on maintaining smooth and efficient movements during each repetition. Some people get worried when they hear the words 'technique' or 'form' mentioned in the gym but remember this is simply

30mins

When running at a pace of 8 kph (5 mph) for 30 minutes a person weighing 56 kg (125 pounds) will burn 240 calories, while for someone weighing 70 kg (155 pounds) it is 298 calories, and at 84 kg (185 pounds) it is 355 calories. Figures are the same for circuit training, while swimming breaststroke burns 300, 372 and 444 calories respectively. For cycling at 19-22 kph (12-14 mph) the calories burnt are 240, 298 and 355. (8)

"Great works are performed not by strength, but by perseverance."

SAMUEL JOHNSON

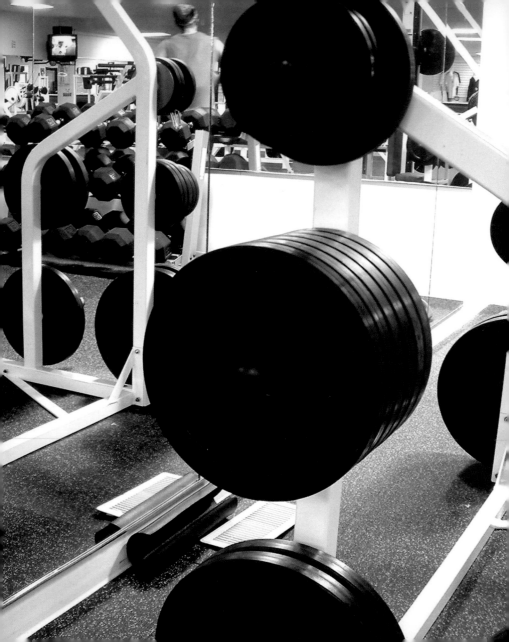

Calories in drinks

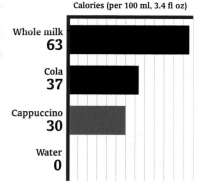

Calories (per 100 ml, 3.4 fl oz)

Whole milk
63

Cola
37

Cappuccino
30

Water
0

It's easy to rack up the calories you consume in drinks each day. Don't cut back and become dehydrated, just balance the type of drinks you enjoy. The chart shows figures for a glass of milk, Coca-Cola and a Starbucks cappuccino with whole milk. (9)

another way of saying 'do the exercise correctly'. Keep your mind focused on the particular part of the body you should be exercising and feel it working during each repetition (eg. with sit-ups actually feel your abs tightening as they pull your upper body up). Focusing in this way helps to keep the other parts of your body working efficiently towards the desired goal (eg. working your abs on sit-ups) and ensures you keep good form. To help keep your muscles loose shake out your limbs one by one and give your neck a gentle roll after completing each exercise.

You might at this stage, especially if you don't feel comfortable with one or more of the exercises, consider booking a session with a personal trainer. Explain what you are doing as the trainer will be able to offer advice on your technique.

If you are one of those keen beans when you start something new, then you will undoubtedly already have bought the latest, flashiest gear your local sports shop had to offer. However, if you are still working out in old shorts and a baggy T-shirt, this is the time to buy some proper training kit (and maybe some basic equipment, such as a mat and an exercise ball, if you've decided you will be following the programme at home). Built-for-purpose kit will make your workouts more comfortable as well as making you feel good about yourself each time you pull it on.

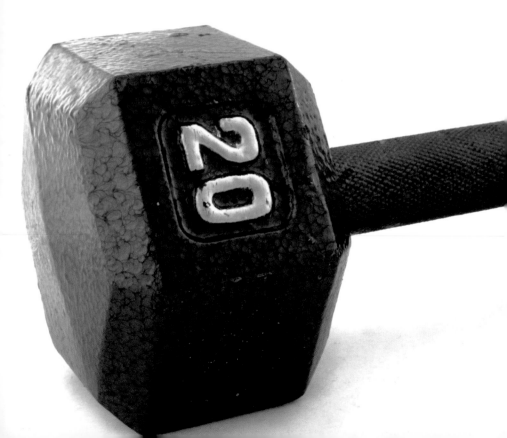

"The difference between a successful person and others is not a lack of strength, not a lack of knowledge, but rather in a lack of will."

VINCE LOMBARDI

that's it!

Week five completed

 Your sessions should be starting to feel more comfortable.

 You know that if you keep doing something you will get better at it. Stick at the exercises.

 Your technique is important. If you are struggling with a particular exercise re-read the instructions on pages 12-15 and consider a session with a personal trainer.

Your should get some basic equipment such as a mat and an exercise ball if you are training at home.

Your notes at the end of the week

week six

Enjoy your healthy life

You've been working hard so now you can enjoy the benefits of feeling fitter…

One of the worst things about being unfit is feeling sluggish. It's a vicious downwards spiral: the more sluggish you feel, the less you feel like exercising and the more unfit you get. And so it goes on. Struggling through the day, always half-tired, becomes the accepted norm. But as you know, and have hopefully rediscovered in the last few weeks, is that it doesn't have to be that way.

Waking up feeling more refreshed and energized (if a little stiff sometimes) is one of the joys of exercising. The day is suddenly something to be attacked and enjoyed with renewed vigour. When the feeling comes, enjoy every minute of it. You've worked hard for it.

We have constantly stressed the need to keep focused on the end goal – your Complete Body Workout challenge – and not to get distracted by other things along the way. So, even if you did take this up to lose a bit of weight or to encourage

YOUR AIM THIS WEEK

Is enjoy the benefits you should already be feeling from exercising. Remain focused on your training and the end goal.

Do not try to force changes in your lifestyle. By concentrating on the end goal you will eventually start to enjoy the other benefits that will come as a by-product of your workouts.

"I'm in a dancing mood. Ya'll know I'm feeling good."

BOB SINCLAIR

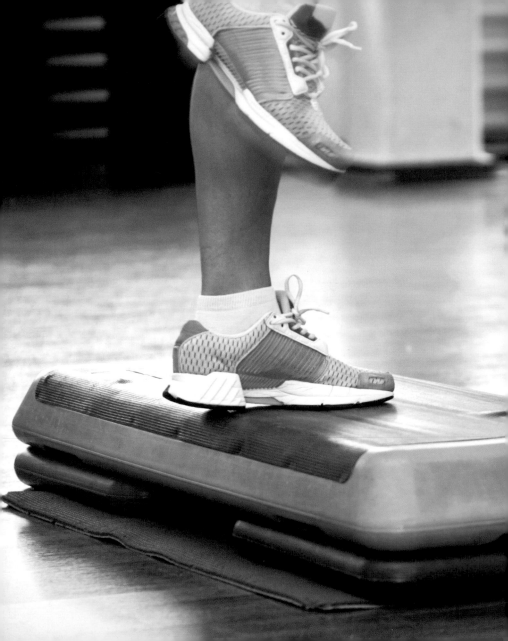

		YOUR DAILY NOTES
MON	5 mins brisk walk, 2 x 20 secs jog with knees up, 1 x sit-ups to max, 1 x 20 stepping alternate lunges.	
TUE	Rest.	
WED	Trial challenge: All to max and with 2 mins recovery. 1 x step-ups for HR recovery test, 1 x press-ups, 1 x sit-ups, 1 x squat on BOSU ball, 1 x front plank.	
THU	Rest.	
FRI	Try a different sport (eg. swimming or cycling), a fun activity (eg. bowling), or go out for a 30 mins walk.	
SAT	Rest. Enjoy another couple of rest days after another good week of exercising.	
SUN	Rest or stretching	

THIS WEEK

 DO – Try to enjoy yourself when you exercise. Believe you can do it and relax.

 CONSIDER – Eating a nutritious breakfast (eg. porridge).

DON'T – Allow yourself to become dehydrated. As you exercise more you will need to start sipping water during exercise breaks.

REWARD

Book an Indian head massage.

yourself to eat better, don't lose sight of what you need to achieve at the end of this 12-week programme. The other benefits will follow in due course, so let them happen naturally.

Your subconscious was set loose the minute you set yourself this goal. Slowly but surely, as you get deeper into the programme, you will notice yourself getting interested in other things such as technique, special kit and so on – and who knows, maybe the weight loss and the better eating habits will follow too. That is the power of setting goals and the power of your subconscious at work.

This doesn't mean you should have expected these few weeks to have transformed yourself into the town's fitness nerd by the way. If you enjoy a glass of wine, it's unlikely your corkscrew has been gathering dust in the cupboard. But maybe you've poured a 'small' instead of a 'large' one once in a while because you are looking forward to the next day's workout and don't want to spoil the enjoyment with a hangover? And if you are a burger lover, it's unlikely the takeaways have become a thing of the past. But maybe you've been tempted by a (healthier) chicken version instead of the usual red meat.

Incidentally, if you don't recognize any of these (or similar) changes in your lifestyle yet there's no need to worry. Always remind yourself that the most positive

5days

Now you have started exercising you are well on your way to meeting guidelines set out by many government health experts – adults aged over 18 should exercise at moderate intensity for 30 minutes at least five days per week. The exercise does not need to be consecutive but should be in bouts of at least 10 minutes at a time. (10)

"Dream as if you'll live forever, live as if you'll die today."

JAMES DEAN

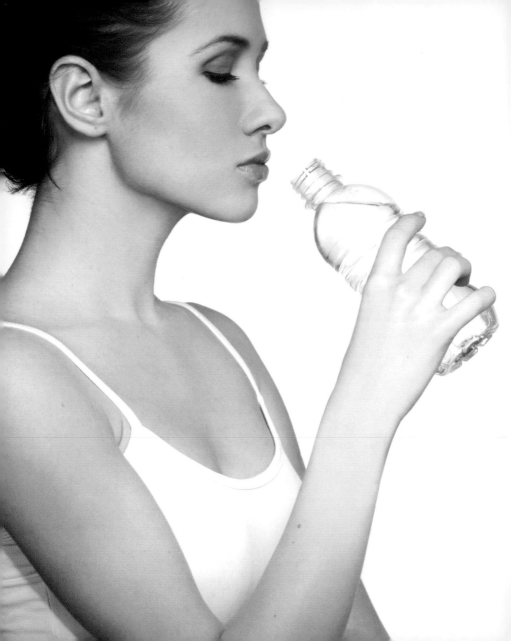

Calories burnt in 30 mins

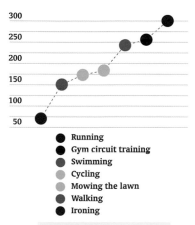

300	
250	
200	
150	
100	
50	

● Running
● Gym circuit training
● Swimming
● Cycling
● Mowing the lawn
● Walking
● Ironing

Different activities use up varying amounts of energy and it's worth noting that even some daily activities help keep you healthy.

The chart shows figures for a walking lawn mower, brisk walking at 6.5 kph (4 mph), moderate cycling at 19-22 kph (12-14 mph), swimming at a pace of 46 metres (50 yards) a minute, and running at 9.5 kph (6 mph). (11)

thing you did was to start this 12-week programme and nothing beats this as a lifestyle change.

This is also the time to start thinking about the details of your challenge day. Try to make an 'event' of it and not to treat it like just another training session, even though it's likely you'll be completing it at home or in the gym you have been training in. You've worked hard for this, so make it a special day. There are a few simple little tricks that can help your mind treat it as a special day. You could buy a new top for the occasion, mark off the day in red letters in your diary, or create a new playlist if you listen to music while you workout. Making an 'event' of it like this will also give you an added spur in the coming weeks.

If you have been using a gym, then try to choose a time when the place is quiet so you won't be disturbed by too many other people during your Complete Body Workout challenge. We've set your challenge day for either Saturday or Sunday (see page 133) to give you a bit of flexibility on this.

If you've got a training buddy you'll be working together on meeting the challenge. If not, then consider asking your partner or a friend to come along to encourage you. It also means you have somebody to go out and celebrate with afterwards – and, who knows, maybe catch up on a glass of that wine you've skipped during training!

"I have not failed.
I've just found
10,000 ways that
won't work."

THOMAS EDISON

that's it!

Week six completed

 You can now enjoy the positive feelings that comes from exercising. Soak up these feelings because you have worked hard.

 You are not trying to change everything in your life but instead concentrating on the end goal.

You know not to worry if you are not seeing or feeling the benefits of your training yet. Keep your enthusiasm levels high and working hard, and you will find that other benefits, such as weight loss, will follow naturally.

 You know it is important to treat your challenge day as an 'event' rather than just another training session.

Your notes at the end of the week

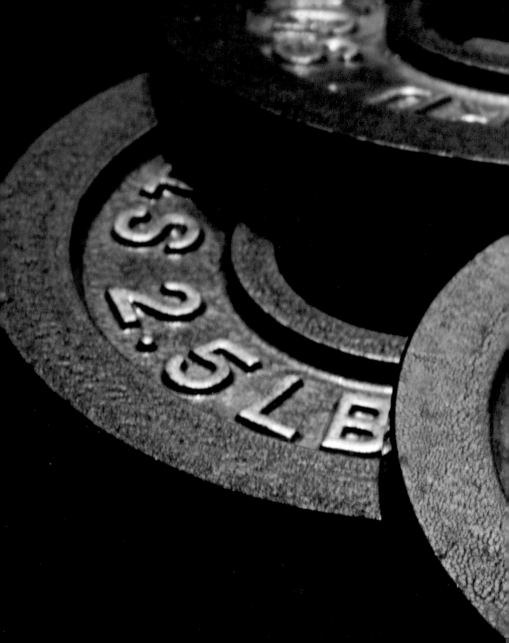

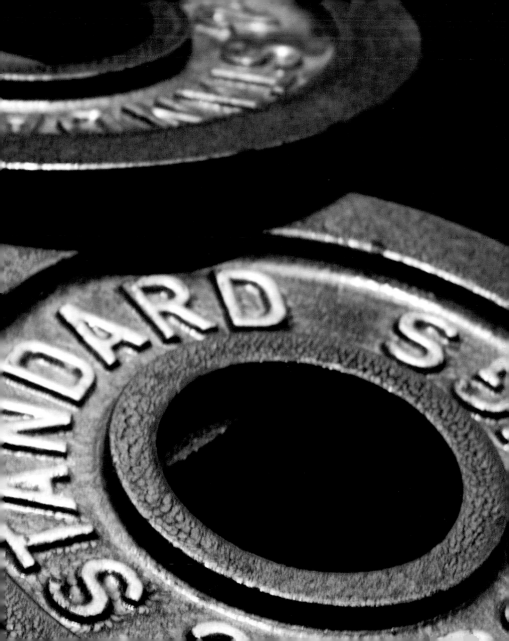

week seven

You're well on your way

Think back and congratulate yourself on how far you have come already…

So here you are at the start of week seven. Did you believe you'd make it this far? Of course you did; it was never in doubt was it? But this is the stage in a training programme when you could start to get the jitters that you haven't done enough work or you are not making progress quickly enough. Some doubts start to creep in. Thoughts like, "I'll never make it," and "What was I thinking starting this?" pop into your head.

All this is perfectly natural because at the start of the programme, 12 weeks seemed a long way away. Now, however, you are well into the training and the end is becoming real.

But this is *not* the time to panic and let your energy or enthusiasm levels drop off. You will already have started to see improvements in your fitness but these first few weeks have really been all about setting a good base from which you can launch yourself towards the end goal. Remember that you were

YOUR AIM THIS WEEK

Is to avoid worrying that you have not done enough training. Just stay focused on the end goal.

The programme and the workouts in it are designed so you will smoothly and successfully progress towards what you set out to achieve at the start. Trust the programme and keep working.

"You can have anything you want if you will give up the belief that you can't have it."

DR ROBERT ANTHONY

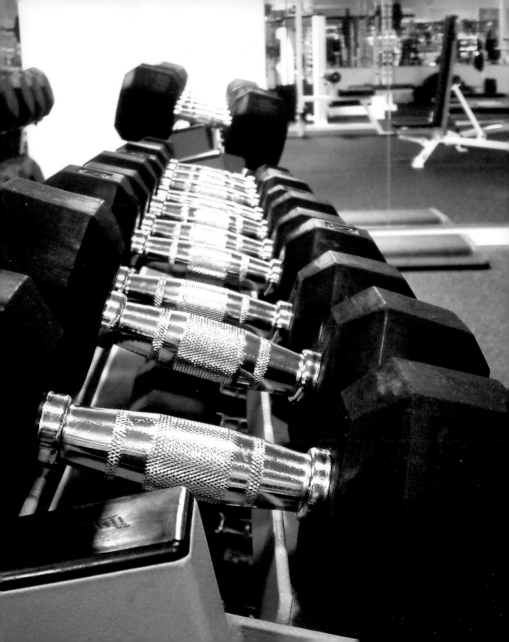

		YOUR DAILY NOTES
MON	5 mins step-ups, 3 x 20 secs jog with knees up, 3 x 15 back raises, 3 x 10 sit-ups, 2 x 12 static lunges (each leg).	
TUE	Rest. Avoid the temptation to do extra sessions on your rest day. Let your body recover properly.	
WED	10 mins stairs, 2 mins jumping jacks, 2 x 12 tricep dips, 1 x 20 stepping alternate lunges.	
THU	Rest.	
FRI	5 mins step-ups, 3 x 20 secs jog with knees up, 3 x 15 back raises, 3 x 10 sit-ups, 2 x 12 static lunges (each leg).	
SAT	Rest. Try to set aside a few minutes for a decent session of stretching today.	
SUN	Rest or stretching.	

THIS WEEK

 DO – Get more active in your daily life, such as walking part of the way to work or using the stairs instead of the lift.

CONSIDER – Your weekly alcohol intake. Alcohol will dehydrate you and lower your energy levels.

DON'T – Start skipping sessions. This is common after a few weeks but consistent training is the only way to get results.

REWARD

Treat yourself to your favourite meal.

out of shape at the start so some basic work was needed. In the next few weeks you will really start to see improvements in your performance. Trust in the programme because it has been carefully designed to gently work you towards your Complete Body Workout challenge.

So have a quiet moment with yourself and celebrate what you have achieved already. Some days are tough, no matter what you do, so accept that as a fact. Other days are good, so look at what you did on these training days and repeat the same thoughts and actions next time you train. Tuck the bad stuff away quickly and keep the good stuff at the forefront of your mind.

Hopefully you have been keeping your notes up to date for each of your sessions and summarizing it all at the end of each week. Writing notes are important for crystallizing your thoughts, and putting them down on paper makes them more concrete. But there is a secondary, and equally important reason for keeping notes. And that is for times like now. Read back over your notes. Allow yourself a wry smile at early comments like, "That was a real struggle," or "It was so tough today, I never knew how unfit I really was!" And restore your enthusiasm levels with the early upbeat stuff like, "I'm tired but I loved every minute of that. Now I want more!" or "This is fun, don't know why I put it off for so long."

7, 8, 9

Most of us grow up being told that we need a 'good eight hours sleep' every night. Experts recommend seven to nine hours sleep a night for an adult – only you will know what is right for you. Try to get into a regular sleep pattern instead of trying to 'catch up' on the weekends as this re-sets your sleep cycle. (12)

"Fitness –
if it came
in a bottle,
everybody
would have
a great body."

CHER

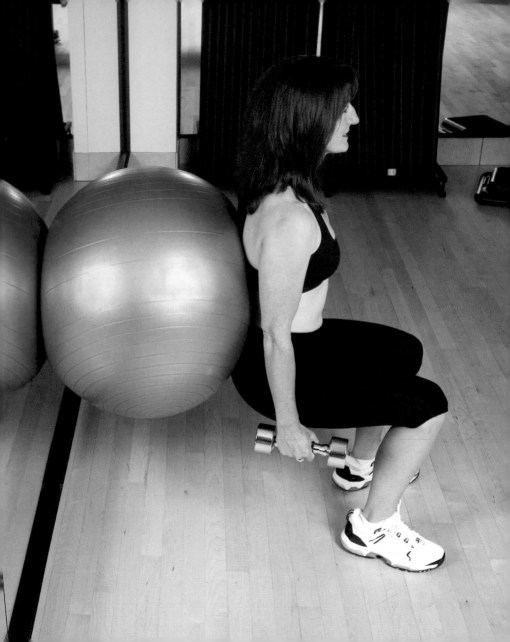

If you have a training buddy you should avoid comparing the progress you are making. By all means push each other along, as it can be healthy, but don't allow this to become a contest. Remember you started out on this challenge for yourself, so don't get caught up in a pointless competition. In particular, you should not let it worry you if your training buddy seems fitter than you at this stage. It is more important that you keep making progress.

Now, how about using your challenge to raise money for a charity? Of course, many of your friends and family should already know you are training hard for your Complete Body Workout challenge so this could be a good opportunity to do something positive for a good cause as well as for yourself. If you do decide to use your challenge to raise some money for charity, this will also help to make the day the special event we encouraged you to make it. Most of us have a charity we support for personal reasons and signing up with your chosen charity will make you more likely to see this challenge through to the end.

Charities welcome support of this kind, so simply fire off an e-mail and explain what you are planning to do. Most charities are geared up to support fundraisers and will have special packs with everything you'll need, such as sponsorship forms, posters, and even security sealed collecting boxes if you want to make use of them.

Health benefits of fitness

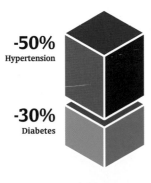

-50%
Hypertension

-30%
Diabetes

Exercising regularly reduces your risk of contracting many chronic diseases. These include Hypertension (50%), Ischaemic heart disease (40%), breast cancer (27%), a stroke (27%). (13)

"For my part I know nothing with any certainty, but the sight of the stars makes me dream."

VINCENT VAN GOGH

that's it!

Week seven completed

 You know there is still plenty of time until your Complete Body Workout challenge so there is no need to worry you are not making enough progress quickly enough.

 You have read back over your notes to remind yourself of the progress you have made already.

You are not worrying if your training buddy seems to be making faster progress than you. Keep focused on what you need to do and not on other people.

You are now past the halfway stage of the programme. You knew you'd get here didn't you? Well done!

Your notes at the end of the week

8 week eight

Recommit to the challenge

It's time to picture the details of a successful conclusion to the programme...

There are now only a few weeks left in your 12-week programme and this is the time to recommit to your goal of a Complete Body Workout challenge. Even though it's less likely than it was at the start, unbelievably some people do still give up after getting this far in a training programme. So to make sure you don't become one of those people (you're surely not even thinking of it are you?) you should reconfirm your commitment.

So we return to day one of the programme when all you had to do was tell five people you were about to embark on a 12-week challenge. Now you need to do it again. It doesn't have to be the same people and it'll be a lot easier this time because it's highly likely that many of your friends and family are following your progress with interest, so they will welcome an update anyway.

However, if you are one of those people who cringes at the idea of talking about yourself and

"The best way to predict the future is to invent it."

ALAN KAY

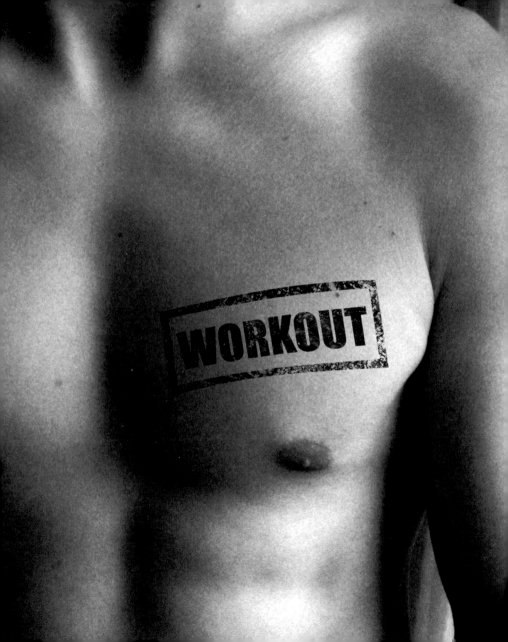

WEEK EIGHT: YOUR TRAINING PROGRAMME AND DIARY

		YOUR DAILY NOTES
MON	5 mins step-ups, 2 x 30 secs jog with knees up, 2 x 20 back raises, 1 x side plank (both sides) to max, 1 x 20 stepping alternate lunges.	
TUE	Rest.	
WED	5 mins up and down stairs, 5 mins jog, 2 mins jumping jacks, 1 x press-ups to max, 2 x 30 leg raises, 2 x 30 squats.	
THU	Rest.	
FRI	5 mins step-ups, 2 x 30 secs jog with knees up, 2 x 20 back raises, 1 x side plank (both sides) to max, 2 x 20 stepping alternate lunges.	
SAT	Rest.	
SUN	Rest or stretching. The next few weeks are crucial for your challenge so make sure you use today to look ahead and make time for your future sessions.	

THIS WEEK

 DO – Analyze the intensity you are working at. You are probably a bit fitter now so you can push yourself a little bit harder, but still keep it easy, it's not the end yet.

CONSIDER – Your vegetable intake. Your body will need the vitamins and minerals in vegetables even more now you are exercising.

 DON'T – Start eating too many snacks. Your appetite will increase as you exercise more but try to choose the healthy option.

REWARD

Time to enjoy your favourite takeaway.

who struggled with this the first time around we appreciate this may be difficult for you. But don't skip this step completely as it is an important part of the overall process.

You certainly do not need to stand on a table in the staff rest room, clap your hands for attention, then declare your commitment in a loud voice to all your colleagues. Well, you can if you wish but they might just think you are on the path to madness not fitness.

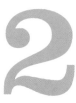

Try to work the subject into the conversation casually. It's easy enough to say to someone: "Sorry, I must go as I am meeting my friend at the gym later. There are only a few weeks to go in that fitness programme I was telling you about a while ago".

One way to raise the subject again is to send round a sponsorship form for your chosen charity. Most people are happy to support a good cause and it will prompt many of them to ask how your training is progressing. Either way, make sure you hear yourself recommitting to the challenge out loud.

This is also a good time to go through the visualization exercise again – this time with a bit more detail added in. There is no doubting the power of the mind and body when working together. Your body may do the work but it is always controlled by

Sports drinks contain two important ingredients – electrolytes (they help your muscles and heart function) and carbohydrates. You can lose electrolytes through very long workouts and the carbohydrates may help provide extra energy. Try sports drinks to see if they are for you, although water will always be important for most active people. (14)

"Promises are like the full moon, if they are not kept at once they diminish day by day."

GERMAN PROVERB

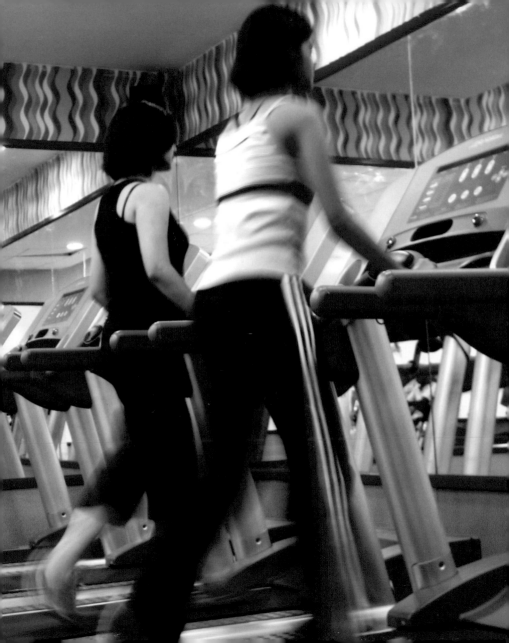

your mind. So let's get your mind to tell your body what it is going to do in a few weeks!

Your goal is already set, and as long as you remain focused on that goal your mind and body will keep working together towards a successful conclusion. You can now help by filling in some of the blanks. Take some time to picture the day of your Complete Body Workout challenge. In your mind 'see' yourself getting ready for the gym, packing your bag with all the things your need – shoes, socks, shorts, wash stuff and so on. Then imagine the gym staff greeting you as you arrive and 'feel' your anticipation as you get changed (maybe into that new top?) and prepare to start. Now picture yourself settling into your first exercise smoothly, maybe hearing the encouragement from your training buddy as your confidence builds.

Then 'see' yourself starting the final exercise (the front plank). You know you are nearly there. If you chose a reward as part of your visualization you should 'remember' the reward (a glass of wine later in the day, perhaps?) when it comes to reward time. This is known as a 'future memory', something you have 'remembered' but which hasn't happened yet! Then let your mind picture you completing your challenge, followed by a call to a supportive friend to let him or her know how you got on. Repeat this exercise as many times as you can in the coming weeks, as it will help you when the actual challenge day arrives.

Calories in alcohol

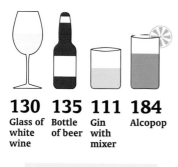

130 **135** **111** **184**
Glass of   Bottle   Gin   Alcopop
white   of beer   with
wine   mixer

On a big night out it's easy to clock up the calories. The graphic shows figures for a 330 ml (11 fl oz) bottle of Stella Artois (4.8% abv), 175 ml (6 fl oz) glass of Jacob's Creek Chardonnay (13% abv), 25 ml (0.8 fl oz) of Bombay Sapphire (40% abv) and mixer, 275 ml (9 fl oz) WKD alcopop. (15)

"Never, never, never give up."

WINSTON CHURCHILL

that's it!

Week eight completed

 You are now well into the second half of this 12-week programme and still going strong.

 You have confirmed your commitment to the Complete Body Workout challenge by updating your friends, family and colleagues on your progress.

 You know your mind and body have been working together towards your goal ever since you set it at the start and they will continue their partnership till the end.

 You have 'seen' the details of your challenge day in your mind. Come the actual day this will help things run smoother.

Your notes at the end of the week

week nine

Maximize your benefits

Revisit all the exercises to see where you can improve...

You already know that – assuming you have the basic technique correct – the more you do an exercise, the more comfortable you will feel with it. But by regularly reviewing your technique for each exercise and improving it where necessary you can make your workouts easier and more enjoyable. Getting your technique right also means you will be getting the maximum benefit from your workouts.

Spend this week looking over the technique notes for all the exercises in this 12-week programme (see pages 4-7), and next time you are working out try to consciously think through each of your movements. Then think back when you have finished and ask yourself if there are any parts of your technique you could improve upon. Try not to become all robotic with your movements (which can easily happen when you break down the individual components) but let your mind and body work together so you can fine-tune your technique without losing the rhythm you have built up already.

YOUR AIM THIS WEEK

Is to spend some time checking through the notes on pages 12-15 and look at areas where you can improve on your own technique.

As you work out, think through each of the movements and afterwards ask yourself where you can change things for the better.

"Exercise should be regarded as tribute to the heart."

GENE TUNNEY

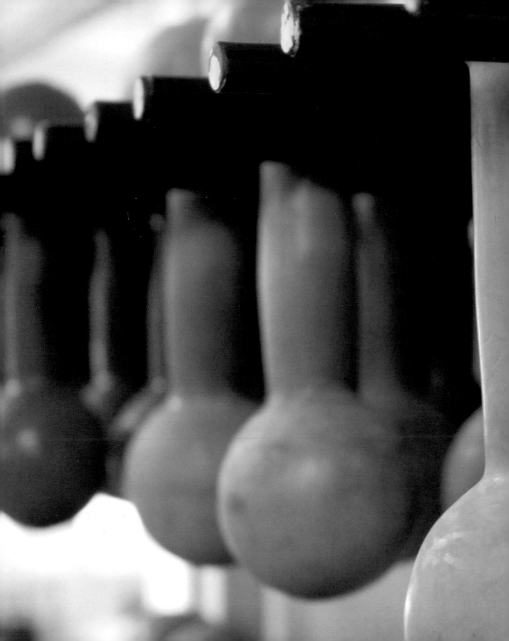

WEEK NINE: YOUR TRAINING PROGRAMME AND DIARY

		YOUR DAILY NOTES
MON	5 mins stairs, 1 min jumping jacks, 45 secs jog with knees up, 2 x press-ups to max, 2 x tricep dips to max, 2 x 20 back raises.	
TUE	Rest.	
WED	5 mins step-ups, 45 secs jog with knees up, 2 x 30 leg raises, 2 x front plank to max, 1 x sit-ups to max.	
THU	Rest.	
FRI	5 mins step-ups, 3 mins jog, 2 x 30 squats, 2 x 15 static lunges each leg, 3 x 20 stepping alternate lunges.	
SAT	Rest.	
SUN	Rest.	

THIS WEEK

 DO – Re-evaluate your technique on each exercise. Remember perfect technique gets better results.

CONSIDER – Joining in group exercises, or finding an exercise partner. It is a lot easier to train with other people

DON'T – Start looking to the finish line yet. You're doing well but there are still a few more weeks of hard work yet.

REWARD

Enjoy a few of your favourite drinks. Watch the hangover!

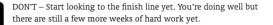

Your Complete Body Workout challenge day consists of five exercises: step-ups, press-ups, sit-ups, squat on BOSU ball and front plank. Pay particular attention to getting these five exercises spot on.

Step-ups are first in the list because they are a great way to warm up your whole body for the exercises ahead (although you should have stretched out your muscles to start with anyway). More than anything step-ups are about building up a nice rhythm (music can certainly help). Start off slowly until you get into your stride and are stepping at the one-leg-per-second pace.

4 or 9

Concentrate on keeping straight and tall, (as if you are trying to impress your former head teacher with your posture) and putting your heel down first as you step up. Once into your rhythm you should be able to feel the power of your legs as they pull you up each time. To help you focus on this try crossing your arms across your chest. Alternatively you may prefer to try holding a small weight in each hand (or a can of beans), as this can help with balance, although be warned, this makes the step-ups even tougher.

Sugars and starches (carbohydrates) found in foods such as pasta, bread, cereal, fruit and vegetables have four calories per gram (0.14 oz) while fat is more than double at nine calories per gram (0.32 oz). Worth knowing when you're trying to get fit and healthy don't you reckon? (16)

You are doing step-ups so you are able to measure your heart-rate recovery. Your heart rate will always go up during exercise but the fitter you are the quicker it will return to normal once you stop. It is important you are able to find your pulse straight

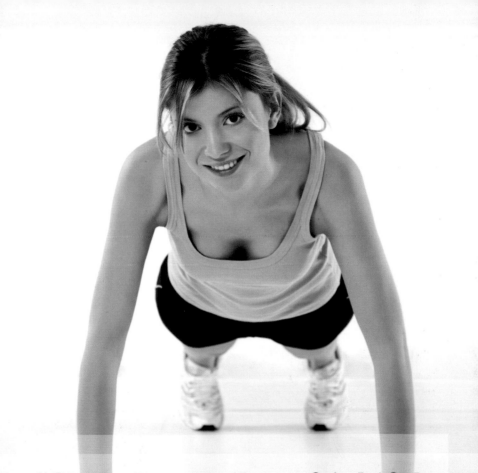

"Obstacles are those frightful things you see when you take your eyes off the goal."

HENRY FORD

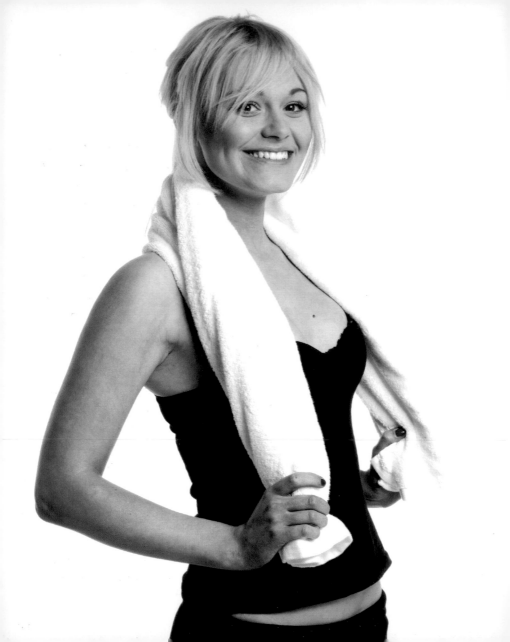

away and not fumble around on your wrist for too long as your pulse changes fairly quickly. If you really struggle then ask a friend to help or even consider buying a heart-rate monitor.

After your two-minute recovery, press-ups are next. It's easy to ignore technique for press-ups because it's such a well-known exercise but remember to pay particular attention to the shape of your back. At all costs avoid using your back muscles to pull yourself up.

As with above, it's easy to become lazy with sit-ups because they are so well known. To get the best from this effective exercise think of pulling your belly button towards your spine. If you really want to test yourself then sit-ups can be done while balancing the base of your back on an exercise ball.

Ah, next up the dreaded leg burning of the squat on BOSU ball! Remember your legs have already been worked with the step-ups so this exercise won't be easy. Keep your back straight and avoid hunching forward. Then take deep breaths and start counting off the seconds.

Back alignment is the key with your final exercise – the front plank. Settle into the position that feels right then push back through your heels as this will straighten up your back. Push back again if you feel yourself losing shape.

A balanced diet

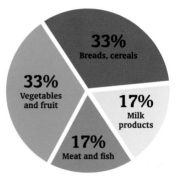

Try to maintain a balanced diet of the 'basic four food groups' in the proportions shown in the chart above and to eat from all of them every day. Also limit the amount of fats you include in your diet. (17)

"A bear, however hard he tries, grows tubby without exercise."

AA MILNE

that's it!

Week nine completed

 You know it is important to build a nice rhythm with step-ups. Start slowly and build up to a pace of one second per leg.

 You know it is easy to ignore your technique when doing press-ups because it is an exercise that is so well known, but you need to concentrate on the shape of your back and avoid sagging.

 You know the squat on BOSU ball is tough and you will feel the dreaded 'leg burn'. Keep your back straight and the seconds will tick by quicker than you think.

 You know the front plank is all about back alignment. Once into position push your heels backs to help straighten your back.

Your notes at the end of the week

week ten

Smoothly does it every time

Keep focused, even if things are going well at the moment…

This exercise thing is getting easy now isn't it? A few weeks ago you could hardly pull on your kit without huffing and puffing, but now here you are, on the verge of completing your challenge. So what's the problem? What can go wrong at this stage?

You might be right. However, you still need to be careful because there are two mind sets that can cause all this hard work to come crashing down, which is why you need to keep your wits about you and stay focused on your goal. One is over-confidence and the other is a lack of self-belief. Which one applies to you – if any – largely depends on your personality, but either could destroy what you are trying to achieve.

Confidence is a good thing, but over-confidence can lead to you doing too much because you start to think you are invincible. Remember you only set out on this programme a few weeks ago, and even if you have made rapid progress (well done by the way), you

YOUR AIM THIS WEEK

Is to keep trusting the programme to see you through to the end successfully.

Do not get over-confident or worry you have not done enough as both of these could lead to you doing extra sessions. Avoid this as extra sessions will only drain your energy.

"By perseverance
the snail reached
the Ark."

CHARLES SPURGEON

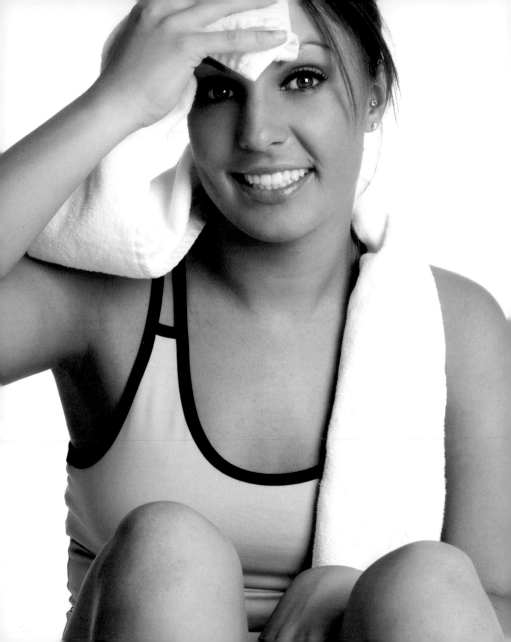

		YOUR DAILY NOTES
MON	5 mins walk up and down stairs, 1 min jumping jacks, 45 secs jog with knees up, 3 x press-ups to max, 3 x tricep dips to max, 3 x 20 back raises.	
TUE	Rest.	
WED	5 mins step-ups, 45 secs jog with knees up, 3 x 30 leg raises, 1 x front plank to max, 1 x side plank (each side) to max, 1 x sit-ups to max.	
THU	Rest. A bit of stretching on your rest day is even more important now you are training so much.	
FRI	5 mins step-ups, 3 mins jog, 3 x 30 squats, 2 x 15 (each leg) static lunges, 2 x 20 stepping alternate lunges, 2 x squat on BOSU ball to max.	
SAT	Rest.	
SUN	Rest or stretching. Ensure you are warm before stretching out your muscles as you have a couple of important weeks ahead..	

THIS WEEK

 DO – Analyze how you feel the day after training. If you are sore you might need to stretch more or check your technique.

 CONSIDER – Taking up a sport or activity you couldn't have done before (when you have completed this challenge!)

 DON'T – Start skipping your warm-ups and cool downs to save time.

REWARD

Have another great cheat day. Eat, drink and be merry.

still need to stick to the plan. This programme has been worked out carefully so you gradually build up your strength and fitness until you are ready for the final day – your Complete Body Workout challenge.

So avoid the temptation to do more than what is set out in each workout and don't do extra sessions when you should be resting. Sometimes, because you are getting a buzz from working out it is tempting to do extra sessions just for the fun of it (or because you feel invincible). If you want to become a gym junkie at a later stage that is fine, but for now stick to the plan or you could burn yourself out or get injured. If you really want to do something extra then use your rest days to do more stretching.

The flip side of this scenario is a lack of self-belief in what you have achieved so far and a fear you are not going to make it. The end result, however, is remarkably similar to over-confidence: you end up doing more sessions than you should. Of course, in this scenario you are doing the extras because you think you need to cram in a bit more, but it is equally as damaging.

A bit like a panicky student who thinks he has not learnt enough, you are tempted to go mad and study through the night as you approach your exam. But the truth, if you have been following the programme, is that you should have little to worry

17-19

> Researchers in Australia and New Zealand found that people who drove after being awake for 17-19 hours performed worse than those who had a blood-alcohol level of 0.5 per cent – the legal limit for drivers in Australia and many European countries. It's not difficult to see that sleep is important for anyone who wants to focus on his/her health and fitness. (18)

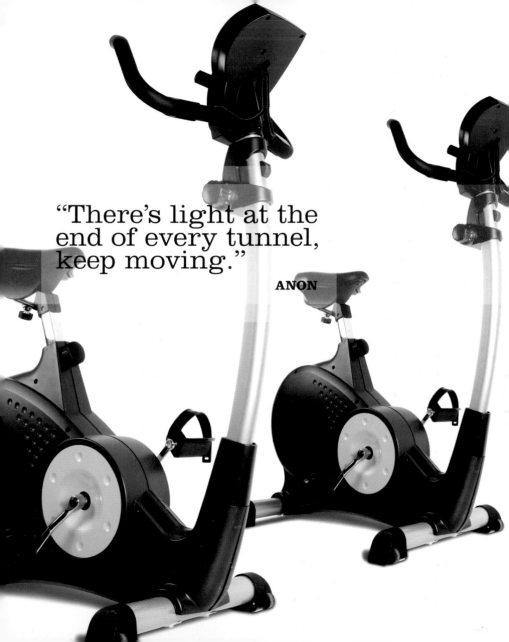

"There's light at the end of every tunnel, keep moving."

ANON

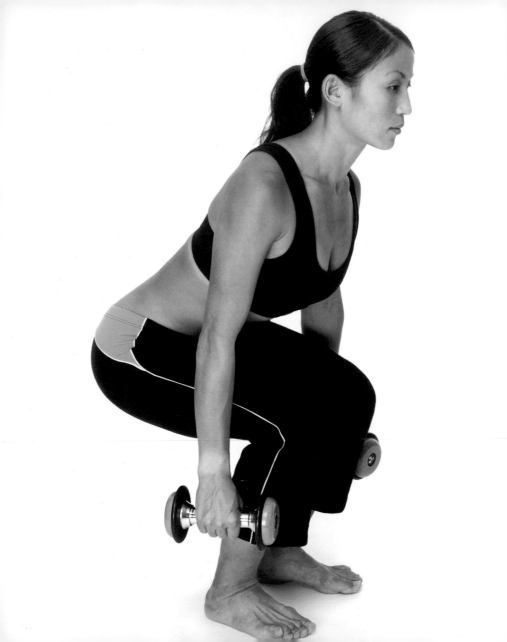

The human body

60%
Water

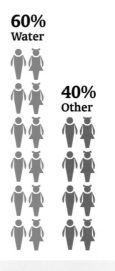

40%
Other

Around 55-60 per cent of your body is made up of water. Your brain is 70 per cent water, blood 83 per cent water and lungs nearly 90 per cent. Make sure you keep yourself topped up by drinking plenty of water throughout the day. (19)

about (of course, if you really haven't done enough then even extra sessions at this stage won't help anyway). All you will do if you try to squeeze in extra sessions at this stage is drain your energy. Just keep focused on good sessions on your workout days and enjoying relaxing days – with a bit of stretching – on your rest days.

Other things that can disrupt your efforts at this stage are sickness or injury. Do everything you would usually do to stay in full health, such as eating and sleeping well, and drinking lots of water during the day. There's nothing more irritating than picking up a niggly cold just as you approach the end of a hard training programme.

When it comes to injuries, you already know that stretching before and after a workout – and on your days off – will help your muscles. Maintain this discipline right to the end.

However, despite all your efforts to stay healthy, sickness or injury may still strike. Don't panic if you have to miss one or two sessions because the base work you have already done will still see you through. It's important you do not continue training if this happens. Under no circumstances should you keep working out through pain. Rest may help but if necessary visit a doctor or physio to get the problem correctly diagnosed and treated.

"When it is obvious that the goals cannot be reached, don't adjust the goals, adjust the action steps."

CONFUCIUS

that's it!

Week ten completed

 You are wondering why you didn't start this earlier. Exercising is starting to become second nature to you.

 You have full confidence in the programme getting you to your end goal – your Complete Body Workout. If you have stuck to the programme you don't need to worry you have not done enough work so avoid the temptation to do extra sessions.

 You know over-confidence, no matter how fit your feel, could also lead to problems. Again, avoid doing extra training sessions just because you are feeling great.

 You will rest and seek professional advice from a doctor or a physio if you fall sick or get an injury. Do not keep training.

Your notes at the end of the week

week eleven

The end is in sight

Now you're so close, start concentrating fully on your challenge…

Professional athletes rarely leave anything to chance as they approach a target they have been training for. All their efforts go into training hard, resting easy and eating as healthily as possible. But they are professional athletes and their whole time is set aside for what they do.

The rest of us living on Planet Reality have to fit in our training and our fitness targets while at the same time juggling work, family, and other commitments. Take your children to school in the morning, get the car to the garage for its annual check-up in time, then off for a full day's work, return mum's call when you get a chance, grab a sandwich and coffee at lunchtime, pick the car up, and oh, don't forget the children now. Phew…

All of this is enough to make a professional athlete go back to bed for a rest just thinking about it. But hang on, you're not a professional athlete so you haven't finished yet. Now you need to get the

YOUR AIM THIS WEEK

Is to realize you can't control everything in your life so, although you want to keep focused fully on the end goal some unexpected events may have to be dealt with.

But you can control some things. This is not the time to start new projects to help distract you.

"First say what you would be and then do what you have to."

EPICTETUS

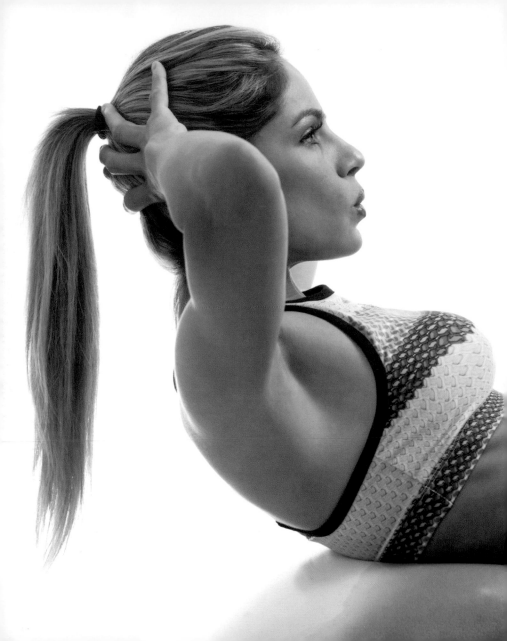

WEEK ELEVEN: YOUR TRAINING PROGRAMME AND DIARY

		YOUR DAILY NOTES
MON	10 mins walk up and down stairs, 2 mins jumping jacks, 45 secs jog with knees up, 3 x press-ups to max, 1 x sit-ups to max, 2 static lunges x 20 (each leg).	
TUE	Rest.	
WED	10 mins brisk walk, 2 mins jumping jacks, 3 x 20 back raises, 3 x 15 sit-ups, 3 x 20 stepping alternate lunges.	
THU	Rest.	
FRI	10 mins walk up and down stairs, 2 mins jacks, 45 secs jog with knees up, 3 x press-ups to max, 1 x sit-ups to max, 2 x 20 static lunges (each leg).	
SAT	Rest. Relax and avoid doing anything stressful because this is your last weekend before the big day.	
SUN	Rest or stretching.	

THIS WEEK

DO – Start to look at your targets. Are they achievable?

CONSIDER – Reading over your notes to remind yourself how far you have come.

DON'T – Panic and think you need to start doing extra training at this stage.

REWARD

Block out a few hours where you can relax and focus on the final week.

family dinner ready, put the children to bed, then hey, maybe you've got a bit of time for your own training at last? That's the reality of keeping fit for most people.

If you think back to why you got out of shape in the first place then one of the main reasons is probably because of pressures on your time (or perceived pressures on your time). It's a common excuse people have for not keeping fit but it's a real one.

You really do have to fight for time to yourself. It's why we have kept the programme short and sharp, and why we recommend that you treat your workouts as appointments by marking them down in your diary or punching them into your phone. But times have changed, so you have made positive steps towards getting fit and have made it a priority to set aside a few minutes, a few times a week, when you can workout.

36°C

Be particularly careful when exercising in hot weather. Once the temperature rises to 36°C (97°F) it is recommended you cancel your session or postpone it to a cooler part of the day as the heat will put a lot of stress on your body. (20)

In short, you are not using time pressures as an excuse not to workout anymore. But let's be honest, there are many things you can't control in your life. If there is deadline at work, you may need to stay in the office late. If someone close to you gets sick, you may need to care for them. You can't control everything. You have to deal with these circumstances the best you can. But there are many things you can control, so let's concentrate on those things.

"Success only comes before
work in the dictionary."

ANON

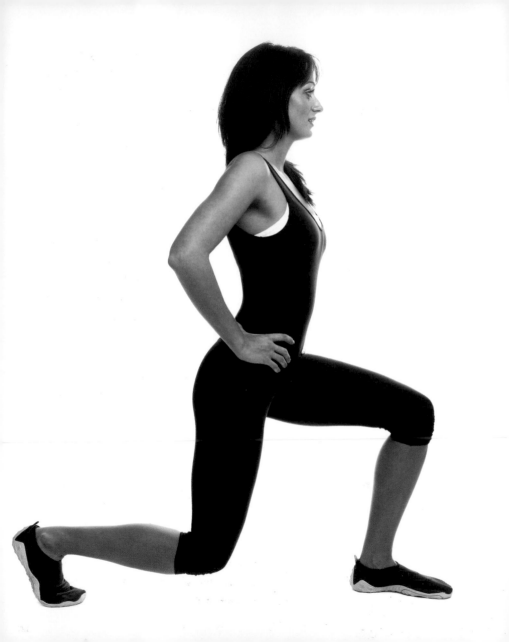

A balanced meal

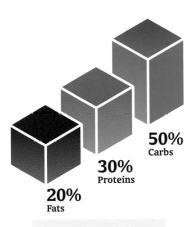

50%
Carbs

30%
Proteins

20%
Fats

Try to balance all food elements with every meal you eat in line with the figures shown in the chart above.

Carbohydrates include rice, bread, fruits and vegetables, proteins come from meat, fish, milk products and eggs, while nuts, avocados, green olives, fish oil and olive oil are a good source of fats. (21)

All of us have those 'to do' lists stored away in our heads (and more than often, in our partner's heads!). But this really is not the time to be dragging out that list and thinking of ticking off a few of them. Come on, if the cupboard in the spare room has not been cleaned out for the last two years, is it really crucial that it needs to be done in the next couple of weeks, just as you approach your Complete Body Workout challenge? We think not.

You may be tempted to get started on tasks like these because you have some nerves as you approach the end of Week 12, but leave that cupboard and all its boxes alone (at least for a couple more weeks till you have finished this challenge)! Nerves can lead to us looking for a distraction and although jobs like this will certainly take your mind off the end goal, they will also drain you physically and emotionally. But come on, why would you ruin all this hard work just to clean out a cupboard?

If you really do need to distract your mind then go for a gentle stroll with your dog, watch a film that motivates you, cook up a new recipe in the kitchen, or get stuck into an easy-to-read book from the best-seller list. At this stage stay focused and avoid anything that makes it harder for you to complete your Complete Body Workout challenge. Instead, keep your mind firmly fixed on what you set out to do a few weeks ago.

"If you have the will to win, you have achieved half your success; if you don't, you have achieved half your failure."

DAVID AMBROSE

that's it!

Week eleven completed

 You know unforeseen problems can crop up in your life at any stage. Acknowledge this happens in life, and work through these problems as calmly as possible.

 You know that although taking on new projects (such as cleaning out the cupboard in the spare room) might distract your mind from the end goal, they will also drain your energy. Avoid!

 You aren't fighting the nerves you may be feeling. Relax and accept this is perfectly normal.

 You know to do something more relaxing – like reading a book – if you really need to distract yourself from your nerves.

Your notes at the end of the week

week twelve

This is it, finally!

You are now ready to complete your challenge successfully...

So, are you ready? Of course you are. You've done the hard work and now you should try to enjoy this week. On Monday you will have your last proper workout – a mini run through of the big day – so go easy and don't push yourself too hard. Otherwise the rest of the week, apart from a brisk walk to keep you loose on Wednesday, should be spent resting, although try to do some stretching.

Don't celebrate just yet because there is still a lot of hard work to do but don't be afraid to wallow in the glow of what is come. You have followed the programme so you *will* succeed with your Complete Body Workout. Remind yourself of this in the next few days.

Make sure you are prepared properly for the day (remember you are trying to make this into an event) and get everything you may need ready ahead of time. Go through the checklist below so you don't forget anything.

YOUR AIM THIS WEEK

Is to enjoy yourself as you successfully finish your Complete Body Workout.

After 12 weeks following this programme you are ready. You have worked hard and nothing can stop you from what you have trained for over these past few weeks.

"All dreams can come true if we have the courage to pursue them."

WALT DISNEY

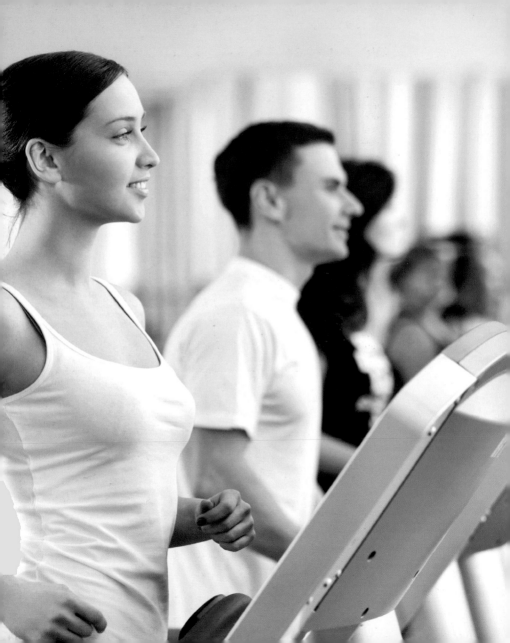

WEEK TWELVE: YOUR TRAINING PROGRAMME AND DIARY

		YOUR DAILY NOTES
MON	2 mins step-ups for HR recovery test, 5-10 x press-ups, 10 x sit-ups, 20 secs squat on BOSU ball, 20 secs front plank (all with 2 mins recovery).	
TUE	Rest.	
WED	Brisk walk for 30 mins.	
THU	Rest.	
FRI	Rest. Try to spend some time stretching.	
SAT	Your Complete Body Workout challenge or rest. Choose the day which is best for you to complete the challenge.	
SUN	Your Complete Body Workout challenge or rest. Choose the day which is best for you to complete the challenge.	

THIS WEEK

 DO – Go for it! Safely challenge yourself and see what you can do.

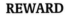 CONSIDER – How you feel at the end of your challenge. What have you achieved already and what more do you want to achieve?

 DON'T – Get disheartened or nervous as you have done well to get this far.

REWARD

Congratulate yourself for your achievement!

Checklist

- ☐ Training shoes
- ☐ Socks
- ☐ Shorts or leggings
- ☐ T-shirt or vest
- ☐ Music
- ☐ Stopwatch
- ☐ Water bottle or sports drink
- ☐ Energy bar
- ☐ Heart-rate monitor (if you are using one)
- ☐ Towel and wet wipes
- ☐ Copy of your Complete Body Workout challenge

The actual night before completing a challenge can often be a bit nervy and it's tough to get a good night's sleep, so try to sleep as well as you can during the rest of the week. On the night before the challenge have a healthy, light dinner, and drink plenty of water so you are well hydrated in the morning. You can make up for lost time afterwards when you are celebrating, but for now, avoid alcohol and caffeine. You may need to go to bed a bit earlier if you have chosen an early-morning start.

Have breakfast and a glass of water an hour (or more) before you start your challenge in the morning. Do not experiment with new foods at this stage – stick to things your stomach has got used to in the training programme. Then, before you set off for the gym, think through what you are about to do.

Try to stick to the schedule you have planned for your Complete Body Workout challenge, even if you are

6-10

If you need a performance boost in the day then a short sleep – or a power nap if you want to sound smart – of just six to 10 minutes could do the trick. If this sounds like something for you then keep the nap short and sharp so you avoid waking up feeling groggy. (22)

"Your goals are the road maps that guide you and show what is possible in life."

LES BROWN

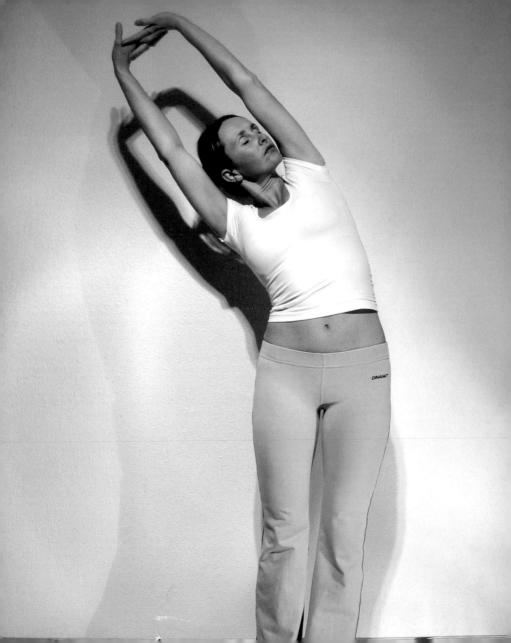

doing your challenge at home. It's easy to put it off or delay it but take this seriously.

If you have had a training buddy for your challenge then chat about the exercises ahead (it'll help calm your nerves) and decide who will be going first. If there are two of you then you may decide to alternate the exercises (so you do one test while your buddy recovers) or you may decide to run through the whole challenge one person at a time. If there are more than two of you then you'll have to take it in turns to complete the whole challenge before the next person starts, otherwise everyone's recovery time will be too long. Draw lots if you can't decide who goes first!

There should be a feeling of anticipation at the start of any challenge like this. Enjoy the buzz at the start, but don't go off too fast on your first exercise – the step-ups. Although this is easy to do when you are nervous or excited, try to keep focused on establishing a steady rhythm, then building up to the one-leg-per-second pace.

If the gym is busier than you hoped, don't panic. Just steadily work through your challenge and keep reminding yourself that you have worked hard and you can do it.

But finally, you are ready… enjoy your Complete Body Workout challenge!

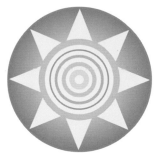

Have you ever noticed how refreshed and good you feel after exercising once the huffing and puffing has stopped?

Numerous studies have found there is a direct link between exercising and feeling happy and satisfied with your life. Getting a smile on your face – can there be a better reason for you to exercise? (23)

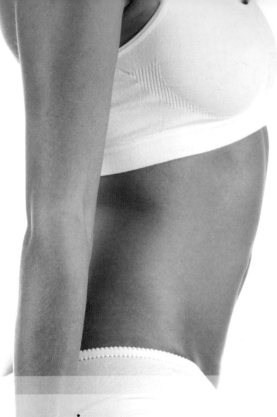

"A person is a success if he gets up in the morning and gets to bed at night and in between does what he wants to do."

BOB DYLAN

that's it!

Week twelve completed

 You have completed your Complete Body Workout challenge in 12 weeks. Well done!

 You can congratulate yourself on what you have achieved in just a few weeks of training.

 You can now enjoy your new-found fitness after 12 weeks of hard work. You worked towards a challenge and you have also made yourself healthier in the process.

 You can celebrate! Choose something you enjoy and reward yourself with it.

Your notes at the end of the week

what now?

Think about your fitness future

**You've completed your Complete Body Workout
challenge. What next…**

After the elation has died down it's possible you may
be feeling a bit flat. This often happens when you
have been working hard towards something and
then you finally complete it. It's not unlike that empty
feeling you get when you return from a long-awaited
trip or a vacation. You've looked forward to it for so
long, then before you know it the whole thing is over.

But this feeling passes soon and is usually replaced
by a renewed enthusiasm to do something new. Of
course, you may not want to do something new. You
may want to renew your close relationship with your
local pizza shop now you have proved to everyone
that you can complete this challenge successfully.
"Right you lot. Will you now shut up? I've shown
you what I can do when I put my mind to it. Now I'm
going back to double cheese and extra pepperoni."
But that really would be a waste don't you think?

You have set a great base for you fitness over the past
few weeks so your training should become easier (it's

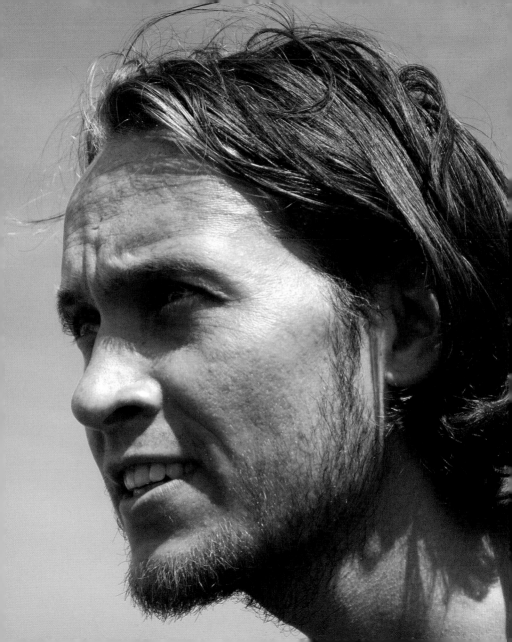

probably a habit already). You've cracked those really tough few sessions in the early weeks, so you are now in a position where you can really push on.

You may be happy with your current level of training and decide to continue with your three, short, sharp sessions a week. This is something you have proved you can manage over the last 12 weeks, something you know you can fit into your lifestyle. If that's your choice then don't be afraid to take a short break (but don't leave it too long) before returning to your three-days-a-week training schedule. Try to vary what you do to avoid boredom, as this is one thing that leads to people giving up.

To make sure this doesn't happen, you should look at introducing some new exercises into your workouts for variation. If you have been following this 12-week programme at home, this may be the time to join a gym, as you'll have more exercises available to you thanks to the range of equipment. If you have been enjoying your sessions as home and want to continue with them, look at buying some of your own equipment. There are only so many things you can do holding a can of beans! You don't need to convert the spare room into a home gym just, yet but a set of weights will expand your options.

You may also consider signing up for a few sessions with a personal trainer. A trainer will introduce you to some new exercises, show you how to do them correctly, as well help to keep you motivated. Most trainers are happy to do sessions for two people at the same time if you ask, so you should be able to train with a friend if this makes you feel more comfortable. For motivation, it would also be an idea to set yourself another target; perhaps devising another Complete Body Workout. A personal trainer can help you work out something specifically geared towards your own (new) fitness levels.

But don't forget there are many other activities you can try such as running, cycling or swimming. All of these will keep you upbeat about keeping fit and you will also start working other muscles in your body.

If you are feeling extra enthusiastic after finishing this programme (and why not?) then a word of warning: while you want to stretch yourself beyond what you have just achieved, don't get too carried away. Remember, one of the reasons you got out of shape in the first place was probably time pressures, so don't suddenly set yourself a target of training six days a week only to find you can't keep up the new schedule. This can lead to frustration and ultimately to you packing it in altogether. You have proved you can fit in three days a week, so it is much better to build up slowly by adding one more day to your training schedule (if that's what you want) and building slowly from there.

First published in 2013 by
New Holland Publishers (UK) Ltd
London • Cape Town • Sydney • Auckland
www.newhollandpublishers.com

A catalogue record for this book is available from the British Library.

ISBN 978 1 78009 232 4

This book has been produced for New Holland Publishers by
Chase My Snail Ltd
London • Cape Town
www.chasemysnail.com

Designer: Darren Exell
Photo Editor: Anthony Ernest
Proof readers: David Chapman, Timothy Shave, Hannah Shipman
Consultant sports psychologist: Russell Murphy
Production: Marion Storz

2 4 6 8 10 9 7 5 3 1

Printed and bound in China by Toppan Leefung Printing Ltd.

The authors and publishers have made every effort to ensure that all information given in this
book is accurate, but they cannot accept liability for any resulting injury or loss or damage to either
property or person, whether direct or consequential and howsoever arising.